Human Muscular Function during Dynamic Exercise

Medicine and Sport Science

Vol. 41

Series Editors   *M. Hebbelinck,* Brussels
R.J. Shephard, Toronto, Ont.

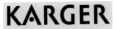

Basel · Freiburg · Paris · London · New York ·
New Delhi · Bangkok · Singapore · Tokyo · Sydney

5th International Symposium on Exercise and Sport Biology,
Nice, France, February 9–11, 1995

Human Muscular Function during Dynamic Exercise

Volume Editors

P. Marconnet, Nice
B. Saltin, Copenhagen
P. Komi, Jyväskylä
J. Poortmans, Brussels

57 figures and 7 tables, 1996

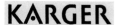

Basel · Freiburg · Paris · London · New York ·
New Delhi · Bangkok · Singapore · Tokyo · Sydney

Medicine and Sport Science

Published on behalf of the
International Council of Sport Science and Physical Education

Founder and Editor from 1969 to 1984
E. Jokl, Lexington, Ky.

Library of Congress Cataloging-in-Publication Data
International Symposium on Exercise and Sport Biology (5th: 1995: Nice, France)
Human muscular function during dynamic exercise / volume editors, P. Marconnet ... [et al.].
(Medicine and sport science: vol. 41)
"5th International Symposium on Exercise and Sport Biology, Nice, France, February 9–11, 1995."
"Published on behalf of the International Council of Sport Science and Physical Education" – T.p. verso.
Includes bibliographical references and index.
1. Exercise – Physiological aspects – Congresses. 2. Muscles – Physiology – Congresses.
I. Marconnet. P. (Pierre) II. International Council of Sport Science and Physical Education. III. Title.
IV. Series.
[DNLM: 1. Muscles – physiology – congresses. 2. Exertion – congresses. W1 ME6490 v.41 1996 / WE 500
I6115h 1996]
QP301.I576 1996
612'.044–dc20
ISBN 3–8055–6274–8 (hardcover. alk. paper)

Bibliographic Indices. This publication is listed in bibliographic services, including Current Contents® and Index Medicus.

© Copyright 1996 by S. Karger AG, P.O. Box, CH–4009 Basel (Switzerland)
Printed in Switzerland on acid-free paper by Thür AG Offsetdruck, Pratteln
ISBN 3–8055–6274–8

Contents

Fatigue and Damage

Preface

Here are the Proceedings of the 5th Nice Symposium on Exercise and Sport Biology. Since 1978, the organizers have been guided by the same motivations: (1) to choose themes and build a program of major interest in the life and health sections of sport science for sport scientists, coaches, physicians, physiotherapists and athletes; (2) to condense the most relevant information into about fifteen conferences over a short period; (3) to propose updated lectures by prominent researchers in basic science as well as data in applied fields by leading experts or new methods and technologies by engineers involved in human machinery; (4) to improve communication among researchers and among laboratory and field teams through extended discussions.

During the past 15 years, sport science has made considerable progress. As a consequence, the number of meetings in the various disciplines (sport biomechanics, sport biochemistry, sport medicine, sport psychology...) has increased in proportion. The aim of the last Nice Symposium was to maintain an integrative view of muscular function through a multidisciplinary approach to the subject of human locomotion.

The 5th Symposium ended with an event of major importance: the foundation of the European College of Sport Science by a group of fifteen senior sport scientists, including sport psychologists and sport sociologists, which indeed extends the integrative function of sport. If the Nice Symposia contributed, even modestly, to the long process that has led to this birth, the organizers will be proud and full of hope for the future of European Sport Science.

The organizers are indebted to the following institutions for encouragement and financial support: Ministère et Direction Régionale de la Jeunesse et des Sports français, Municipalité de Nice, Université de Nice-Sophia-Antipolis, Conseil Général des Alpes-Maritimes, Conseil Régional de la région PACA. The staff, whose work contributed strongly to the success of the meeting, deserves special mention.

P. Marconnet, Nice

Marconnet P, Saltin B, Komi P, Poortmans J (eds): Human Muscular Function during Dynamic Exercise. Med Sport Sci. Basel, Karger, 1996, vol 41, pp 1–9

....

Effects of Shortening Velocity and Oxygen Consumption on Efficiency of Contraction in Dog Gastrocnemius

Pietro E. di Prampero, Johannes Piiper

Department of Biomedical Sciences, University of Udine, Italy, and
Max-Planck-Institut für Experimentelle Medizin, Göttingen, Deutschland

Introduction

In frog sartorii anaerobically stimulated at 0–10 °C, the mechanical work performed per mole ATP split (w*P) is on the order of 8 kJ mol^{-1} (and the shortening speed is maximal) when the ATP concentration is equal to the value prevailing at rest. With decreasing ATP concentration, w*P increases (and the velocity of shortening decreases) to attain about 22 kJ mol^{-1} (and about 30% of maximal velocity) when the ATP concentration is reduced to about half the value at rest [1–3]. Similar considerations apply to the dog gastrocnemius at 37 °C stimulated anaerobically during blood flow occlusion, the only difference being that in dog gastrocnemius w*P is larger: 14 and 28 kJ mol^{-1}, for ATP concentrations of 100 and 50% of resting value, respectively [4, 5]. It is possible to calculate from these data that the thermodynamic efficiency of ATP splitting increased from ~ 0.3 to ~ 0.5 with decreasing ATP concentration from 100 to 50% of the values at rest [2, 3, 5].

These observations suggest that, in anaerobic conditions, the principal determinant of the velocity of shortening of the muscle is the ATP concentration: as this last decreases, and the muscle approaches exhaustion, the speed decreases. In these conditions, however, the work performed per mole ATP split, and the thermodynamic efficiency of muscle contraction, increase. Thus, slower shortening velocities are associated with a more efficient transformation of chemical into mechanical energy, a fact that should indeed be expected on purely theoretical grounds [6]. From the point of view of the external power output, this state of affairs is advantageous since the decreased speed of shortening is compensated for, at least in part, by a concomitant increase of w*P. Indeed, since the effective power output depends on the shortening speed and on w*P, the increase of the latter permits to maintain an optimal power output over a larger speed range than would otherwise be the case [7].

We shall briefly consider the mutual relationships between O_2 consumption ($\dot{V}O_2$), mechanical power output (w), overall efficiency (ϕ) and velocity of contraction (v) during aerobic rhythmic work in dog gastrocnemius. The data were obtained and published in the mid-sixties [8, 9]; in the present study they will be analysed under a different angle

Methods

The muscle preparation has been previously described in several papers [4, 8, 9] to which the reader is referred for further details. Suffice it here to say that, in anaesthetised dogs, the gastrocnemius plantaris muscle group (about 0.1 kg average wet mass) was isolated from the surrounding tissues and its main vein cannulated. The tendon was severed and attached to a spring exerting a constant force of 80 N (i.e. about 40% of maximal isometric force). The displacement of the proximal end (close to the tendon) of the spring was recorded at each contraction by means of a potentiometer, whereas the force of the spring was monitored by a strain gauge at its distal end. The muscle was stimulated, via its centrally cut motor nerve, with short trains of impulses of 1 ms duration and supramaximal voltage and tetanic frequency (about 40 Hz). The duration of each tetanus (0.2 s) was such as to permit a nearly complete shortening (about 80% of maximum) while keeping the static part of the contraction to a minimum. Each tetanus was followed by a pause of 2.8 s, so that the frequency of the tetani was 20 per minute. The stimulation period lasted 8–10 min and was repeated 4–5 times on each muscle group with 30 min interval between working periods. At the end of the experiment, the animal was sacrificed with a massive dose of chloralose urethane.

Throughout each stimulation period, the following parameters were measured: (1) venous outflow, which in this preparation is essentially equal to the blood flow through the muscle [8,9]; (2) arteriovenous differences in O_2, CO_2 and lactate contents, (3) mechanical work performed at each contraction, as given by the constant load (80 N) times the corresponding shortening, and (4) maximal velocity (v) during the shortening phase of the tetanus. This allowed us to calculate: (i) steady-state $\dot{V}O_2$ and to express it in watts on the basis of the observed respiratory quotient (the average RQ was 0.86, for which the energetic equivalent of O_2 is 20.5 J ml^{-1}); (ii) the mechanical power, as given by the mechanical work per contraction times the frequency of the tetani, and (iii) the overall mechanical efficiency (ϕ), as given by the ratio w $\dot{V}O_2^{-1}$. These data were measured several times during the stimulation period to make sure that a steady state was attained. The lactate output from the muscle was also assessed to verify that the muscle was indeed working aerobically.

Statistical Analysis

In the present study, all correlations between variables were calculated by least squares analysis of linear or linearized functions. It was shown by Brace [10] that when both variables are subject to essentially unknown errors, as is the case in the present conditions, standard

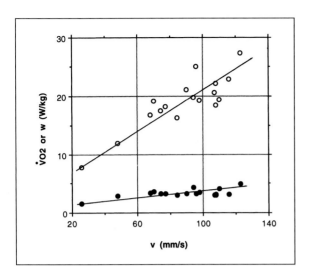

Fig. 1. Oxygen consumption ($\dot{V}O_2$, ○) and mechanical power (w; ●), in W kg^{-1} are plotted as a function of the maximal velocity of shortening (mm s^{-1}). Straight-line regressions are described by: $y = 3.37 + 0.178x$ ($R^2 = 0.76$) for $\dot{V}O_2$ and $y = 0.81 + 0.029x$ ($R^2 = 0.40$) for w ($n = 17$).

least squares analysis underestimates the slope of linear regressions. In these conditions, the best estimate of the slope (A) is equal to the slope found by conventional analysis, divided by the correlation coefficient and the intercept if found from the mean values of y and x: $B = \bar{y} - A\bar{x}$. Throughout this study, slopes and intercepts of linear, or linearized, regressions are calculated as suggested by Brace [10].

Results

The experimental results showed that: (1) O_2 consumption ($\dot{V}O_2$) and (2) mechanical power output (w) increased approximately linearly with the velocity of shortening (fig. 1). However, for a given increase of v, the increase of $\dot{V}O_2$ was relatively larger than that of w, this resulting in (3) a slight decrease of efficiency (see fig. 3). These data are presented under a different angle in figure 2 where the contraction velocity is plotted as a function of the difference between $\dot{V}O_2$ and w. The data of figure 2 are interpolated by a power function:

$$v = 2.85 \, (\dot{V}O_2 - w)^{1.24} \tag{1}$$

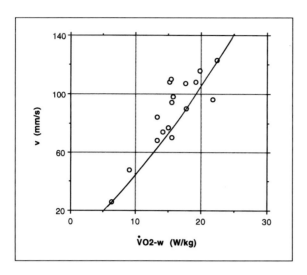

Fig. 2. Velocity of shortening (v, mm s^{-1}) is plotted as a function of the difference between steady-state oxygen consumption and mechanical power ($\dot{V}O_2$–w, W kg^{-1}). Regression is described by: y$=2.85$x$^{1.243}$ (R$^2=0.85$; n$=17$).

(n$=17$; R$^2=0.85$; p<0.001) which yielded a substantially higher determination coefficient (R^2) than all other tested functions (linear, 0.74; exponential, 0.74; logarithmic, 0.78, 2nd- or 3rd-order polynomial, 0.79).

Discussion

Equation 1 and figure 2 show that the velocity of contraction is closely associated with the difference between $\dot{V}O_2$ and the mechanical power output. Thus, even if no empirical relationship can be taken for proof of underlying causal mechanisms, the difference between $\dot{V}O_2$ and w, which is a measure of the chemical power dissipated by the system, can be viewed as the driving force controlling the velocity of muscle shortening, an important variable indeed, if the muscle has to do any amount of work in a time shorter than infinity. Therefore the dissipated power should not be considered a mere waste, even if it necessarily leads to a decreased efficiency of contraction (see below).

The power function interpolating the data of figure 2 has been drawn on purely empirical bases. However, regardless of its underlying physiological significance (if any), equation 1 shows that the overall mechanical efficiency depends on both v and $\dot{V}O_2$: an increase of v leads to a decrease of efficiency, whereas an increase of $\dot{V}O_2$ leads to an increase of efficiency. The few lines that follow will be devoted to make explicit the above statement.

Equation 1 can be expressed in logarithmic form:

$$\log v = \log a + b \log(\dot{V}O_2 - w), \tag{2}$$

where $\log a \ (= \log 2.85) = 0.46$ and $b = 1.24$. Since

$$w = \phi \ \dot{V}O_2 \tag{3}$$

replacing equation 3 into equation 2 and re-arranging, one obtains:

$$\log \dot{V}O_2 + \log(1 - \phi) = (\log v - \log a)b^{-1}. \tag{4}$$

Leaving the term containing the quantity ϕ to the left side, taking the antilogarithm, rearranging and replacing the constants a and b with their numerical values, one obtains:

$$\phi = 1 - 10^{(-0.37 + 0.80 \log v - \log \dot{V}O_2)}. \tag{5}$$

Equation 5 shows formally what was stated above, i.e. that the efficiency of contraction depends both on the speed of shortening and on O_2 consumption: and increase of v leads to decreased efficiency, whereas an increase of $\dot{V}O_2$ is associated with an increased efficiency.

Equation 5 also shows that, for any given $\dot{V}O_2$, the relationship between efficiency and v is univocally set: four such ϕ/v functions have been calculated, for $\dot{V}O_2$ values of 10, 15, 20, and 25 W kg^{-1}: they are plotted in figure 3, together with the experimental values of ϕ and w. The iso-$\dot{V}O_2$ functions of figure 3 show that an increase of velocity without a concomitant increase of $\dot{V}O_2$ would rapidly lead to impossibly low values of efficiency. The experimental data show that $\dot{V}O_2$ does indeed increase substantially with increasing v (fig. 1), the result being that ϕ decreases only slightly over a five fold range of velocity. This, coupled with the increase of $\dot{V}O_2$ mentioned above leads to a continuous rise of the mechanical power output (albeit at a decreasing rate) over the entire range of contraction velocities (fig. 3).

The observed increase of efficiency with increasing $\dot{V}O_2$, for a given shortening velocity can presumably be explained as follows: under aerobic conditions, an increase of $\dot{V}O_2$ is necessarily associated with, and presumably due to, a decrease of phosphocreatine and to a minor extent of ATP concentrations in muscle [5, 8, 11]. In turn, this is associated with a more efficient transformation of the chemical energy of ATP hydrolysis into mechanical energy of shortening [3].

During aerobic work at steady state, the efficiency of muscle contraction (ϕ) can be viewed as the product of the efficiencies of: (i) transformation of

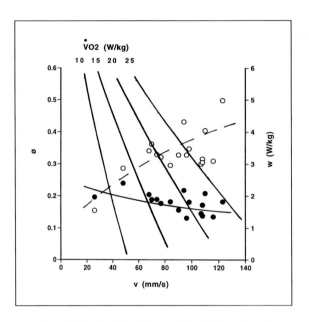

Fig. 3. Mechanical efficiency (ϕ; ● left ordinate) and mechanical power (w, ○, right ordinate) are plotted as a function of the maximal velocity of shortening (mm s^{-1}). Iso-$\dot{V}O_2$ lines are also drawn, as from equation 5 (see text for details).

the free energy of ATP into mechanical energy (ϕs) and (ii) ATP resynthesis at the expense of oxidative phosphorylation (ϕr):

$$\phi = \phi s \, \phi r, \tag{6}$$

where the suffixes s and r stand for splitting and resynthesis. Equation 6 can also be written in a different way, i.e., for a single mole of reaction:

$$\phi = w*P \, n/\Delta H*O_2 \tag{7}$$

where $\Delta H*O_2$ is the enthalpy change per mole of O_2 consumed and n is the number of moles of ATP resynthesized per mole of O_2 consumed [5].

For an average RQ = 0.86, as in the present experiments: (1) $\Delta H*O_2 = 461.4$ kJ mol^{-1} and (2) 6 moles of ATP are resynthesized per mole of O_2 consumed, i.e. n = 6 [5]. It can therefore be calculated from equation 7 that w*P ranged from 17 kJ mol^{-1} (for $\phi = 0.22$) to 11.5 kJ mol^{-1} (for $\phi = 0.15$).

The molar free energy change of ATP hydrolysis ($\Delta G*ATP$), for a given pH, M^{2+} concentration and ionic strength is given by:

$$\Delta G*ATP = \Delta G* \circ ATP + RT \, \ln([ATP])([ADP \, P_i])^{-1} \tag{8}$$

Table 1. Four representative values of oxygen consumption ($\dot{V}O_2$, W kg^{-1} wet muscle mass) and shortening velocity (v, mm s^{-1}), ranging from the highest to the lowest observed in this study, are reported together with the corresponding estimated values of work performed, free energy change and thermodynamic efficiency of ATP splitting (w*P and ΔG*ATP, kJ mol^{-1}, ϕATP)

$\dot{V}O_2$, W kg^{-1}	10	15	20	22
v, mm s^{-1}	40	63	94	120
w*P, kJ mol^{-1}	17.0	14.6	13.1	11.5
ΔG*ATP, kJ mol^{-1}	50.0	49.0	47.0	45.0
ϕATP	0.34	0.30	0.28	0.26

where $\Delta G^* \circ ATP$ ($= RT \ln K^{-1}$) is the value applying at standard 1 *M* concentrations. If the concentrations of phosphocreatine (PC), ATP, and ADP are known, ΔG*ATP can be calculated from equation 8, assuming that: (i) the nucleotides are in equilibrium at the muscle level: PC + ADP = ATP + creatine (Cr) and ATP + AMP = 2 ADP, the corresponding equilibrium constants being Keq = 20 and Keq = 0.4, respectively [12]; (ii) $\Delta G^* \circ ATP = 30$ kJ mol^{-1}, which is strictly true for pH = 6.90, T = 273 °K and pMg^{2+} = 2 − 3 [13]; (iii) the unbound ADP, in equilbrium with the other nucleotides is only 10% of the biochemically determined ADP concentration [12], and (iv) the inorganic phosphate concentration $[P_i]$ amounts to $P_i = Cr + 1.5$ [5]. This set of assumptions, together with the concentrations of PC, ATP, ADP and Cr, determined under similar experimental conditions [8], allowed us to calculate ΔG*ATP. It is reported in table 1 for four $\dot{V}O_2$ values from the lowest to highest observed in this study, together with the corresponding values of w*P, velocity of shortening and thermodynamic efficiency of ATP splitting.

These data show that also under aerobic conditions w*P and the thermodynamic efficiency of ATP hydrolysis decrease with increasing $\dot{V}O_2$ and speed of shortening. Even so, however, the decreased overall efficiency is more that compensated for by the increased $\dot{V}O_2$. As a consequence, the mechanical power output keeps increasing with $\dot{V}O_2$ and shortening speed, albeit at a decreasing rate (fig. 3.).

The data discussed so far were obtained on isolated dog gastrocnemii stimulated to rhythmic isotonic aerobic work. In this muscle group, the axis of the individual fibres forms an angle (angle of pennation) with the axis along which the muscle shortens. As a consequence, the speed of shortening of the fibres is not equal to that of the muscle as a whole, but depends on the angle of pennation. In turn, this may vary from one muscle to the other, thus increasing the scatter of data, without however altering the physiological significance of the observed phenomena. In addition because of the supramaximal type of stimulation (see Methods), the muscle works as a whole and the reasons why, in different experimental periods on the same muscle, and/or in different muscles, $\dot{V}O_2$, shortening velocity and mechanical power varied as described above remained unexplained. As such, these data are difficult to apply to exercising humans, in which conditions the metabolic power generation, the speed of muscle shortening and the mechanical power output are controlled modulating the number and type of motor units recruited and the frequency of discharge of the corresponding motoneurons.

Nevertheless, it is tempting to compare the present experimental conditions to the situation applying during all-out efforts in man. In this case, the rapid fall of the ATP stores, initially brings about a substantial increase of efficiency which is probably enough to compensate for the decreased velocity of contraction which is also brought about by the ATP fall. As the efforts proceed, however, a limit is rapidly reached, after which this tradeoff between (decreasing) speed of shortening and (increasing) efficiency is not possible any more. If this is indeed so, the effective power output may then decrease below that required to continue the effort, thus bringing the exercise to a stop or to a substantial decrease in power. These considerations may also help explaining why only about half the high-energy phosphates stores of the muscle can be utilised at maximal power during very strenuous exercise in man [14].

Finally, the preceding discussion emphasizes an additional reason, beyond that of permitting a sudden burst of high intensity 'anaerobic alactic' efforts [5], underlying the high PC concentration observed in skeletal muscles of all mammalian species, and of many other species as well. Indeed, because of the equilibrium constant of the creatine kinase reaction, a high PC concentration permits to keep [ATP] relatively high and stable over a wide range of metabolic rates, in spite of the corresponding larger decreases of [PC] [8]. Thus, w*P and the overall efficiency of work performance remain low. As a consequence, the difference $\dot{V}O_2 - w$ ($= \dot{V}O_2 (1 - \phi)$) is high enough to permit a substantial velocity of shortening.

In conclusion, in a world moulded by the competition between prey and predator, evolution by natural selection seems to have given priority to speed rather than to economy. Alternatively, the emergence of a system where speed was given priority over economy made the prey-predator competition a powerful tool for directing evolution.

References

1 Chaplain RA, Frommelt B: The energetics of muscular contraction. I. Total energy output and phosphorylcreatine splitting in isovelocity and isotonic tetani of frog sartorius. Pflügers Arch 1972; 334:167–180.

2 Kushmerick MJ, Davies RE: The chemical energetics of muscle contraction. II. The chemisty and power of maximally working sartorius muscles. Proc R Soc Lond B 1969;174:315–353

3 di Prampero PE, Boutellier U, Marguerat A: Efficiency of work performance and contraction velocity in isotonic tetani of frog sartorius. Pflügers Arch 1988;412:455–461.

4 di Prampero PE, Meyer M, Cerretelli P, Piiper J: Energy sources and mechanical efficiency of anaerobic work in dog gastrocnemius. Pflügers Arch 1981,389:257–262.

5 di Prampero PE, Energetics of muscular exercise. Rev Physiol Biochem Pharmacol 1981;89:143–222.

6 Wilkie DR: Thermodynamics and the interpretation of biological heat measurements. Progr Biophys Biophys Chem 1960;10:260–298

7 di Prampero PE: Shortening speed and muscular efficiency. From frog muscle to exercising man; in Wieser W, Gnaiger E (ed): Energy Transformations in Cells and Organisms. Stuttgart, Thieme, 1989, pp 46–53.

8 Piiper J, di Prampero PE, Cerretelli P:Oxygen debt and high energy phosphates in gastrocnemius muscle of the dog. Am J Physiol 1968;215:523–531.

9 di Prampero PE, Cerretelli P, Piiper J. Energy cost of isotonic tetanic contractions of varied force and duration in mammalian skeletal muscle. Pflügers Arch 1969;305:279–291.

10 Brace RA:Fitting straight lines to experimental data. Am J Physiol 1977;233: R94–R99.

11 di Prampero PE Margaria R: Relationship between O_2 consumption, high energy phosphates and the kinetics of the O_2 debt in exercise. Pflügers Arch 1968;304:11–19.

12 Canfield P, Maréchal G: Equilibrium of nucleotides in frog sartorius muscle during an isometric tetanus at 20°C. J Physiol 1973;232:453–466.

13 Curtin NA, Gilbert G, Ktretzschmar, KMK, Wilkie DR: The effects of performance of work on total energy output and metabolism during muscular contraction. J Physiol 1974;238:455–472.

14 Margaria R, di Prampero PE Aghemo P, Derevenco P, Mariani M: Effect of a steady state exercise on maximal anaerobic power in man. J Appl Physiol 1971;30:885–889.

Prof. Pietro E. di Prampero, Department of Biomedical Sciences, University of Udine,
Via Gervasutta 49, I–33100 Udine (Italy)

Marconnet P, Saltin B, Komi P, Poortmans J (eds): Human Muscular Function during Dynamic Exercise. Med Sport Sci. Basel, Karger, 1996, vol 41, pp 10–20

··························

Human Power Output – Determinants of Maximum Performance

Anthony J. Sargeant

Department of Muscle and Exercise Physiology, Vrije University, Amsterdam, The Netherlands

Introduction

In human locomotion, the ability to sustain and generate mechanical power output is of fundamental importance. In order to examine those factors which influence power output, we developed an isokinetic cycle ergometer system [1–3]. Using this experimental approach, we were able to measure power generated by the main locomotor muscles at movement frequencies and hence shortening velocities which are realistic in terms of human locomotion. Technically, the system has the merit that in this constrained form of exercise it is relatively easy to measure the forces generated at the foot-pedal interface and to control the pedalling rate. The latter aspect is crucial since even though we measure power produced by the whole leg hip complex and not individual muscles, it is still necessary to take account of the 'global' power velocity relationship of the active musculature [4].

Maximum Power in Short-Term Exercise

Using this system, a series of investigations have indicated that maximum peak power is achieved in this cycling exercise at a pedalling rate of about 120 rev/min (fig. 1). An important issue that needs to be addressed however is whether subjects can achieve maximal activation of muscle voluntarily in this repetitive dynamic exercise. We believe that the consensus of evidence indicates that complete (or nearly, $>95\%$) complete activation can be generated voluntarily. Evidence to support this view comes from studies where electrical

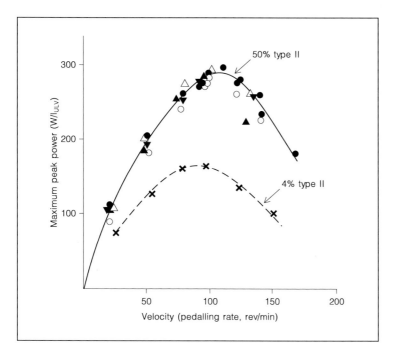

Fig. 1. Relationship of maximum peak power to pedalling rate. Power is standardised for upper leg muscle volume (ULV). Data for 5 subjects, with 50% type II fibres are given. For comparison data are given for an ultra-marathon runner with only 4% type II fibres present [group data from Sargeant et al., 1]. Figure reprinted with permission from Sargeant [12].

stimulation has been applied to human muscle during dynamic contractions [e.g. 5, 6].

Contribution to Power from Different Muscle Fibre Types

In maximally activated 'mixed' muscles such as the human knee extensors all muscle fibre types might be expected to make a contribution to maximum power output (except in the unlikely event that the maximal velocity of shortening of the slowest fibres were exceeded: see Sargeant and Beelen [7] for reasons why this is unlikely). The implications for power output from 'mixed' human muscles which have fibre populations with different force velocity characteristics can be illustrated by reference to a simplified model (fig. 2, 3). In this model, type I and type II fibre populations are treated as two discrete populations with maximum velocities of shortening (V_{max}) in the ratio of 1:4 and each with the same shape force velocity relationship (a/P_o constant). In fact, the reality is that there is a continuum of properties across the fibres,

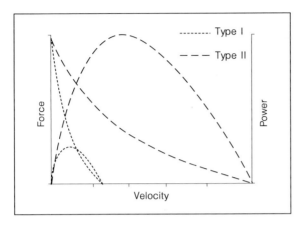

Fig. 2. Force and power in relation to velocity for a slow (type I) and a fast (type II) population of fibres which have the same specific force but V_{max} in the ratio 1:4 (note the very low power generated by the type I compared to type II fibres. Reprinted with permission from Sargeant and Beelen [7].

for example, in the V_{max} due partly to the fact that many human fibres co-express different proportions of the myosin heavy-chain isoforms, which are important determinants of the contractile properties of the fibres [8–10]. Nevertheless, if we assume in a mixed muscle that there is a summation of the power output from equal proportions of type I and II fibres this will give the combined power velocity relationship shown in figure 3. We can then relate this *combined* power to locomotor velocities by reference to the earlier observation that maximum power in cycling exercise is attained at about 120 rev/min. From this it can be seen that type I fibres may be operating at their optimum velocity for maximum power output (V_{opt}) at a pedalling rate of $\sim$60 rev/min while many of the type II fibres (based on the *mean* value used in the model) will have an optimum velocity well in excess of that seen in normal locomotion. As previously discussed, these implications from the model seem reasonable [7, 11] and as also indicated by the data for an ultramarathon runner with only a very few type II fibres in his vastus lateralis muscle (fig. 1).

Mechanical Efficiency and Sustaining Power Output

If little is known for certain regarding the power/velocity relationships of different human muscle fibres, even less is known about the mechanical efficiency/velocity relationships. On the basis of animal experiments, we have specu-

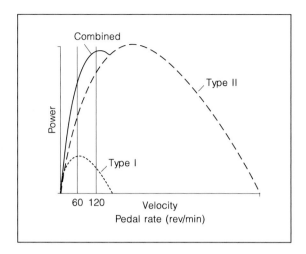

Fig. 3. The component and combined power velocity relationship for a whole muscle (modelled as if composed of two discrete populations of fibre types present in equal proportions, see text). The superimposed pedalling rates are derived by reference to the group data in figure 1. Reprinted with permission from Sargeant and Beelen [7].

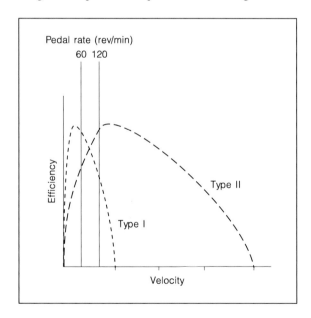

Fig. 4. Schematic of the possible relationships between mechanical efficiency and velocity for the modelled fibre types. In the absence of systematic data, no relative difference between the maximum efficiencies is given – each type is normalised to the same maximum. The velocity range equivalent to pedalling rates of 60–120 rev/min is derived from figure 3. Reprinted with permission from Sargeant and Jones [11].

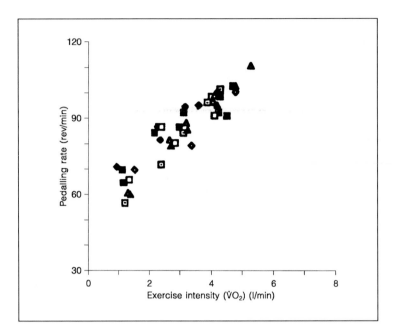

Fig. 5. Relationship between the freely chosen pedalling rate and exercise intensity for a group of 8 trained cyclists riding their own bicycles at different constant speeds (20–47 km/hr). Reprinted with permission from Sargeant [12].

lated that the mean for human type I and II fibres may be of the form shown in figure 4 [11]. One consequence would be that at some intermediate velocity ($\sim$90 rev/min in the figure), the mechanical efficiency of the fibre types would be identical. In addition, within the locomotor range (that is 60–120 rev/min) there is a reciprocal change in the efficiencies. The hierarchical pattern of recruitment implies that at low levels of exercise type I fibres would be primarily recruited with a progressive increase in the type II fibre recruitment as the intensity of exercise increased. This would suggest that if the proposed relationship shown in figure 4 is correct then there should be a progressive increase in the optimum pedalling rate for overall maximum efficiency as exercise intensity increases. In fact when experienced cyclists were asked to select their own gear, and hence pedalling rate, when cycling at different constant speeds around an indoor arena this is precisely what they did (fig. 5). It might also be noted that world record holders for the world 1-hour cycling record, which is very high intensity sustained exercise, have average pedalling rates of $\sim$105 rev/min [12].

There are however many difficulties in relating measurements made at the whole body level to events in the muscle fibres. These include problems relating to: the pattern of muscle fibre population recruitment; the interaction between changes in velocity of contractions with the frequency and duration of the contractions; the estimation of the proportion of energy turnover dissipated in moving the limbs rather than performing mechanical work on the ergometer; and also to the fact that the mechanical efficiency at the muscle level is labile – as may be indicated by the observation of a slow component to oxygen uptake kinetics at high-intensity exercise, an effect which, contrary to much standard teaching, results in a marked curvilinearity of the oxygen uptake/power output relationship in whole-body cycling exercise (fig. 6) [13].

Plasticity of the Neuromuscular System

The neuromuscular system demonstrates considerable plasticity. Metabolic and contractile properties of skeletal muscle fibres can be altered both in the long term (chronic plasticity) and in the short term ('acute' plasticity).

Chronic Plasticity
Experimental interventions, such as cross-innervation or chronic stimulation, have been shown to elicit profound changes in the properties of animal muscles [e.g. 14–16]. Although there have been many investigations using chronic stimulation in animals, there have been relatively few in humans, and the effects elicited have been less dramatic and evidence for changes in myosin isoform expression equivocable [e.g. 17]. Similarly, while training programmes based on voluntary activation have been shown to increase fatigue resistance, it has again been difficult to demonstrate changes in myosin expression. It may be that in both cases there is not usually a significant enough departure from the normal 'background' activity.

'Acute' Plasticity
Muscle fibre properties can be transformed acutely – most notably by exercise itself. It has been shown in animal experiments that the effect of fatigue on the force velocity relationship is to reduce both isometric force generation and the maximum velocity of shortening (V_{max}). As a consequence of the latter change, there is a much greater loss of maximum power than would be expected from the loss of isometric force alone (fig. 7) [18]. Analogous experiments in whole-body human exercise also indicate an increasing loss of power as the velocity of contraction increases [3] (fig. 8).

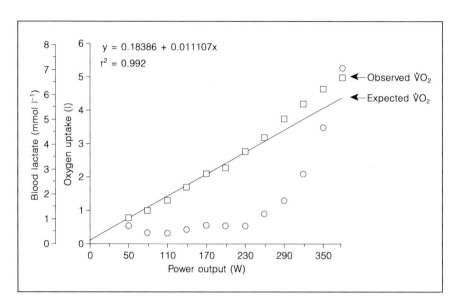

Fig. 6. Oxygen uptake (□) and blood lactate (○) in relation to power output. Note the curvilinear VO_2/power output relationship. Subject AK pedalling at 100 rev min^{-1}. VO_2 is the mean of the last minute of each 3-min increment of power output. Blood for lactate concentration was sampled at the end (3 min) of each increment. The linear regression was calculated from the VO_2/W data below the stage at which a sustained increase in blood lactate was observed. Reprinted with permission from Zoladz et al. [13].

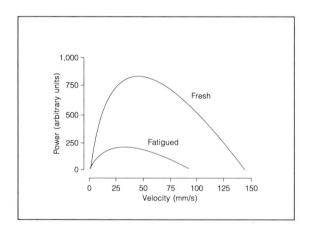

Fig. 7. Power (arbitrary units) in relation to velocity for fresh and fatigued rat medial gastrocnemius muscle. Note: in the fatigued muscle isometric force was reduced to ~50% but power to ~25% of the value for fresh muscle due to the additive effect of the decrease in V_{max}. Based on data from De Haan et al. [18].

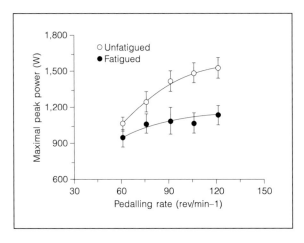

Fig. 8. Human maximum peak power cycling at 5 different pedalling rates in fatigued and unfatigued states. Mean ($\pm$SE) data for 6 subjects. Reprinted with permission from Beelen and Sargeant [3].

Exercise may also lead to potentiation of power output – most dramatically as a consequence of an increased muscle temperature – whereby there is transformation of the muscle to faster properties (fig. 9) [19]. Thus the *acute* transformation of muscle to slower properties consequent upon high-intensity fatiguing exercise may be obscured by the effect of the metabolic heat of that exercise leading to an increase in muscle temperature and a transformation of the muscle to faster characteristics [3, 20].

Growth and Age Effects on Human Power

Specific muscle power that is power appropriately normalised for muscle volume appears to be lower in children and adolescents than in adults although there are difficulties in making accurate measurements of muscle size in the intact human [for a review see Sargeant, 21]. However, since similar observations have been made in young rats where muscle mass can be precisely measured, this does appear to be a real phenomenon [22]. The underlying mechanism is not clear, it may be hormonal in origin or it may be related in some way to rapid increases in muscle fibre length.

In old age there is some evidence for a transformation of muscle towards slower characteristics. This may be the consequence of the reported loss of

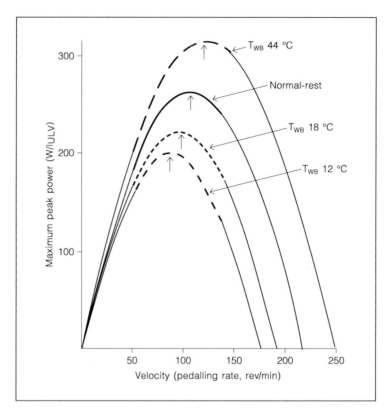

Fig. 9. The relationship of maximum peak power during isokinetic cycling and pedalling rate. Power is expressed as watts per litre of upper leg muscle volume (ULV). Data are given for normal resting conditions at room temperature and following 45-min immersion in water baths at 44° C, 18° C and 12° C. Limits of the experimental data are given by thicker sections of the lines. Arrows indicate the optimum velocity which increases with temperature. Adapted from Sargeant [19].

large motor neurones [23, 24]. The process of denervation and re-innervation by sprouting from the remaining smaller motor neurones may lead to a conversion to slower properties and 'clumping' of the fibres belonging to one motor unit. There is also some suggestion that there is an increase in the number of fibres co-expressing larger proportions of slower myosin heavy-chain isoforms indicating a transformation at the molecular level [25]. Such changes although tending towards causing a loss of fine motor control might not present serious functional problems although maximum power would be reduced. If however there were other changes–including for example muscle atrophy, a greater predisposition to damage and a slowing of subsequent regeneration, as well as colder muscles due to poorly vascularized limbs–power-generating capability may fall below critical thresholds for daily activities [12].

References

1   Sargeant AJ, Hoinville E, Young A: Maximum leg force and power output during short-term dynamic exercise. J Appl Physiol 1981;51:1175–1182.
2   Sargeant AJ, Dolan P: Effect of prior exercise on maximal short-term power output in man. J Appl Physiol 1987;63:1475–1482.
3   Beelen A, Sargeant AJ: Effect of fatigue on maximal power output at different contraction velocities in humans. J Appl Physiol 1991;71:2332–2337.
4   Beelen A, Sargeant AJ, Wijkhuizen F: Measurement of directional force and power during human submaximal and maximal isokinetic exercise. Eur J Appl Physiol 1994;69:1–5.
5   Beelen A, Sargeant AJ, Jones DA, de Ruiter CJ: Fatigue and recovery of voluntary and electrically elicited dynamic force in humans. J Physiol 1995;484:227–235.
6   James C, Sacco P, Jones DA: Loss of power during fatigue of human leg muscles. J Physiol 1995; 484:237–246.
7   Sargeant AJ, Beelen A: Human muscle fatigue in dynamic exercise; in Sargeant AJ, Kernell D (eds): Neuromuscular Fatigue (Academy Series). Amsterdam, Royal Netherlands Academy of Arts and Sciences/North Holland, 1993, pp 81–92.
8   Larsson L, Moss RL: Maximum velocity of shortening in relation to myosin isoform composition in single fibres from human skeletal muscles. J Physiol 1993;472:595–614.
9   Sant'Ana Pereira JA de, Wessels A, Nijtmans L, Moorman AFM, Sargeant AJ: New method for the accurate characterisation of single human skeletal muscle fibres demonstrates a relation between mATPase and MyHC expression in pure and hybrid fibres types. J Muscle Res Cell Motil 1995; 16:21–34.
10 Ennion S, Sant'Ana Pereira JA, Sargeant AJ, Young A, Goldspink G: Characterisation of human skeletal muscle fibres according to the myosin heavy chains they express. J Muscle Res Cell Motil 1995;16:35–43.
11 Sargeant AJ, Jones DA: The significance of motor unit variability in sustaining mechanical output of muscle; in Gandevia S, Enoka RM, McComas AJ, Stuart DG, Thomas CK (eds): Fatigue, Neural and Muscular Mechanisms. New York, Plenum Press 1995; pp 323–338.
12 Sargeant AJ: Human power output and muscle fatigue. Int. J. Sports Med 1994;15:116–123.
13 Zoladz JA, Rademaker A, Sargeant AJ: Oxygen uptake does not increase linearly with power output at high intensities of exercise in humans. J Physiol 1995;488:211–218.
14 Buller AJ, Eccles JC, Eccles RM: Interactions between motoneurones and muscles in respect of the characteristic speeds of their responses. J Physiol 1960;150:417–439.
15 Salmons S, Vrbová G: The influence of activity on some contractile characteristics of mammalian fast and slow muscles. J Physiol 1969;201:535–549.
16 Pette D, Vrbová G: Adaptation of mammalian skeletal muscle fibres to chronic stimulation. Rev Physiol Biochem Pharmacol 1992;120:115–202.
17 Rutherford OM, Jones DA: Contractile properties and fatiguability of the human adductor pollicis and first dorsal interosseous: A comparison of the effects of two chronic stimulation patterns. J Neurol Sci 1988;85:319–331.
18 De Haan A, Jones DA, Sargeant AJ: Changes in power output, velocity of shortening and relaxation rate during fatigue of rat medial gastrocnemius muscle. Pflügers Arch 1989;413:422–428.
19 Sargeant AJ: Effect of muscle temperature on leg extension force and short-term power output in humans. Eur J Appl Physiol 1987;56:693–698.
20 Rademaker A, Zoladz JA, Sargeant AJ: Muscle temperature and short-term power output following prolonged exercise in humans. J Physiol 1994;479:51P.

21 Sargeant AJ: Short-term muscle power in children and adolescents; in Bar-Or O (ed): Advances in Pediatric Sports Sciences. Champaign, Human Kinetics Publishers, 1989, vol 3, chapt 2, pp 41–63.

22 Lodder MAN, de Haan A, Lind A, Sargeant AJ: Changes in morphological and functional character-istics of male rat EDL muscle during growth. J Muscle Cell Contractil 1993;14:47–53.

23 Campbell MJ, McComas AJ, Petito E: Physiological changes in ageing muscles. J Neurol Neurosurg Psychiatry 1973;36:174–182.

24 Doherty RJ, Vandervoorts AA, Taylor AW, Brown WE: Effects of motor unit losses on strength in older men and women. J Appl Physiol 1993;74:868–874.

25 Klitgaard H, Zhou M, Schiaffino S, Betto R, Salviati G, Saltin B: Ageing alters the myosin heavy chain composition of single fibres from human skeletal muscle. Acta Physiol Scand 1990;140:55–62.

Prof. A.J. Sargeant, Department of Muscle and Exercise Physiology, Vrije University,
Van der Boechorstraat 9, NL–1081 BT Amsterdam (The Netherlands)

Marconnet P, Saltin B, Komi P, Poortmans J (eds): Human Muscular Function
during Dynamic Exercise. Med Sport Sci. Basel, Karger, 1996, vol 41, pp 21-31

....

Efficiency in Repeated High-Intensity Exercise

J. Bangsbo

Copenhagen Muscle Research Centre, August Krogh Institute,
University of Copenhagen, Denmark

Introduction

Mechanical efficiency during submaximal exercise has received much attention. Less is known about energy turnover during supramaximal exercise and in particular during repeated intense exercise. Various human studies have, however, focused on the metabolic response during high-intensity intermittent exercise [1–4]. When repeating ten 6-second sprints on a cycle ergometer, Gaitanos et al. [4] found a 27% reduction in mean power output, whereas the glycogenolytic and glycolytic rates during the tenth sprint were only 10 and 13% of the rates during the first sprint. Similar findings were obtained when 30-second maximal isokinetic cycling bouts were repeated at 4-min intervals [3]. The work performed during the third exercise was 82% of that achieved during the second exercise bout, but the glycogen utilization and lactate accumulation were reduced by 68 and 31%, respectively. The creatine phosphate (CP) and adenosine triphosphate (ATP) breakdown were similar for the two exercises. With the same exercise model, the subjects in a study by McCartney et al. [2] carried out four sprints. It was observed that the glycogen concentrations at the end of the last three sprints were similar, indicating a lowering in glycogenolysis when the exercise was repeated.

These studies suggest that the energy turnover per work unit is lowered when intense exercise is repeated. However, the aerobic energy production was not determined and the work output decreased during the exercise, which makes it difficult to relate the metabolic changes to the development of force. Furthermore, for various reasons the total anaerobic energy production could not be accurately quantified (see below), which is important if energy production during supramaximal exercise (represents exercise intensities higher than an intensity eliciting maximum oxygen uptake) is to be determined. Therefore, before discussing energy production during repeated intense exercise, it will be considered how the anaerobic energy production may be quantified. In the last section the use of the oxygen deficit as a measure of the anaerobic energy production will be discussed, since the oxygen deficit method is frequently used and the topic is closely related to energy production during intense exercise.

Quantification of Energy Turnover during Intense Exercise

In several studies, muscle biopsies have been obtained before and after muscle contractions in order to quantify the anaerobic energy production during intense dynamic exercise [for a review, see ref. 5]. Based on the decrease in muscle CP and ATP, as well as on accumulation of metabolites like pyruvate and lactate, the anaerobic energy production of the biopsied muscle has been determined. This kind of determination leads to an underestimation of the energy production by the muscle, since the energy turnover related to the release of lactate to the blood from the exercising muscles, which may represent a substantial contribution to the total anaerobic energy production [6], is not taken into account. Furthermore, it is difficult to determine the total anaerobic energy turnover during whole-body exercise, such as cycling, from measurements on biopsies from a single muscle as the mass and the activity of the muscles involved are unknown and as the metabolic response of the biopsied muscle may not be representative of all the muscles included. This led us to use another model in which subjects are performing knee-extensor exercise in a supine position. It has the advantage that the exercise is confined to the quadriceps muscle and thus, the mass of the active muscle can be determined fairly precisely. Furthermore, blood flow to the exercising muscle can be measured and venous blood draining the exercising muscle can be collected.

The knee-extensor model was used to examine the anaerobic energy production during intense exercise. Subjects performed approximately 3 min of exhaustive exercise at a work rate corresponding to an energy production of about 130% of peak $\dot{V}O_2$ for the exercising muscles [6]. Arterial and femoral venous blood samples were collected and leg blood flow was measured frequently during the exercise. In addition, a muscle biopsy was taken before and immediately after the exercise. The net lactate production by the quadriceps muscle, determined as the sum of total lactate release [taking into account that lactate was taken up by the hamstrings/adductor muscles during the knee-extensor exercise; see ref. 7] and lactate accumulation, corresponded to an energy production of 69 mmol ATP · kg^{-1} w.w. By adding the energy released from muscle CP breakdown, changes in nucleotides, and accumulation of glycolytic intermediates, the total anaerobic energy production was estimated to be 91 mmol · kg^{-1} w.w. This was slightly higher than the anaerobic ATP provision of about 76 mmol · kg^{-1} w.w. by a quadriceps muscle after 200 s of intermittent electrical stimulation [8]. The difference was probably caused by the occlusion of the circulation in the latter study. In support of this is the finding that the lactate released to the blood during the one-legged dynamic exercise corresponded to an anaerobic energy production of 23 mmol · kg^{-1} w.w. [6].

Leg oxygen uptake of the active muscles was also measured during the exhaustive knee-extensor exercise. It amounted to 550 ml · kg^{-1} active muscle. To this should be added the O_2 bound to Mb in muscle and Hb in blood, and further O_2 dissolved in the muscles, which corresponds to about 11 ml · kg^{-1} w.w. [5]. Thus, the total oxygen utilization was around 560 ml · kg^{-1} or 124 mmol ATP · kg^{-1} w.w. Combined, the aerobic and anaerobic energy production was 215 mmol ATP · kg^{-1} w.w. or 17.2 mmol ATP · kg^{-1} · kJ^{-1}.

The one-legged knee-extensor model seems to allow for an accurate quantification of the energy production during dynamic exercise in an isolated muscle. It was therefore used in a series of studies examining energy turnover and mechanical efficiency during repeated intense exercise.

Energy Turnover during Repeated Intense Exercise

In one knee-extensor study, an exhaustive exercise bout was repeated shortly (2.5 min) after high-intensity intermittent exercise, and exercise time was reduced from 3.73 to 2.98 min [9]. Lactate production during the second exercise was markedly lowered, whereas ATP and CP utilization was similar. Thus, the anaerobic energy production was significantly reduced also when expressed per work unit (fig. 1). During the second exercise leg $\dot{V}O_2$ was slightly elevated, but could not compensate for the lowered anaerobic energy production from glycolysis. Thus, the total energy turnover per work unit was lower during the second exercise (fig. 1). In another experiment, subjects repeated exhaustive knee-extensor exercise after 1 h of passive recovery [10]. Exercise duration was 12% shorter during the second bout compared to the first. Lactate production was reduced with 40% whereas anaerobic and total energy production per unit of work was lowered by 22 and 10%, respectively (fig. 2).

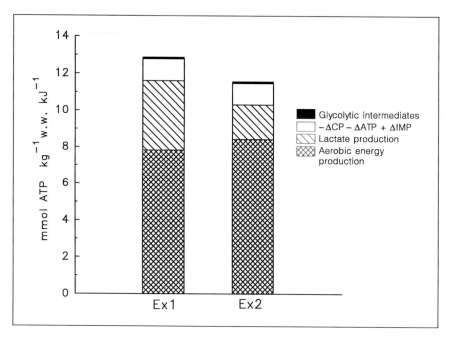

Fig. 1. Total muscle energy production expressed per unit of work (mmol ATP · kg^{-1} w.w. · kJ^{-1}) estimated as the sum of aerobic energy production and anaerobic energy production determined as energy release related to net lactate production, utilization of ATP, creatine phosphate and accumulation of IMP as well as accumulation of glycolytic intermediates during two exhautive knee-extensor exercise bouts (Ex1 and Ex2) separated by 16 min of intense intermittent exercise. Ex1 significantly different ($p < 0.05$) from Ex2.

The findings in these knee-extensor studies suggest that the mechanical efficiency is elevated when intense exercise is repeated. Findings in other studies using *dynamic* exercise are in line with this suggestion (see Introduction). It is also in accordance with the observation by Sahlin and Ren [11] that the energy cost per unit force was reduced by 30% when an intense exhaustive *isometric* contraction was repeated after 2 min of recovery.

In order to evaluate whether the reduction in energy production was constant during the entire second exercise period, another study was performed in which subjects repeated exhaustive one-legged knee-extensor exercise after a 4-min recovery period. On one day they exercised with the left leg for 20 s at a constant power output (62.9 ± SE 2.9 W). After 30 min of rest they performed two exhaustive exercise bouts (62.9 ± 2.9 W) with the right leg separated by 4 min of rest. On another day, subjects exercised with the left leg to exhaustion at the same power output as the first day (62.9 ± 2.9 W)

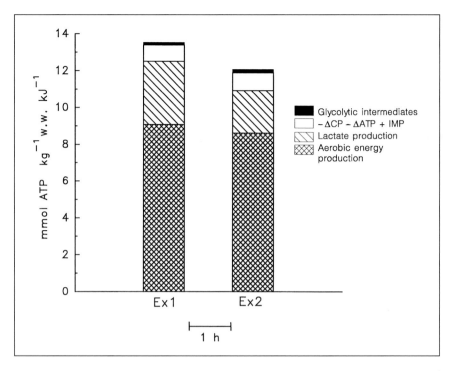

Fig. 2. Total muscle energy production expressed per unit of work (mmol ATP · kg^{-1} w.w. · kJ^{-1}) estimated as the sum of aerobic energy production and anaerobic energy production determined as energy release related to net lactate production, utilization of ATP, creatine phosphate and accumulation of IMP as well as accumulation of glycolytic intermediates during two exhaustive knee-extensor exercise bouts (Ex1 and Ex2) separated by 1 h of rest. Ex1 significantly different ($p < 0.05$) from Ex2.

followed by a 4 min recovery period and a 20-second exercise bout. A muscle biopsy was obtained prior to and immediately after each exercise bout. Basically, the experimental design was so that the metabolic response could be evaluated after 20 s and at exhaustion of two exhaustive exercise bouts separated by 4 min. The mean duration of the first exercise bout was 148 ± 54 s, which was 47% longer ($p < 0.05$) than for the second exercise period. Lactate accumulation and estimated anaerobic energy production were reduced ($p < 0.05$) by 69 and 36%, respectively, during the first 20 s of the second exercise bout compared to the first bout (fig. 3); [Bangsbo et al., to be published]. During the remaining part of the second exercise the mean rate of anaerobic energy production and energy production per work unit were the same for Ex1 and Ex2 (fig. 3). These findings suggest that it is mainly in the

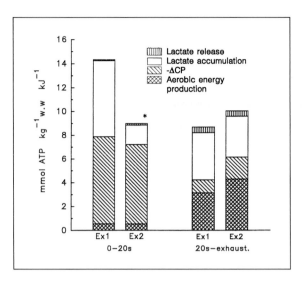

Fig. 3. Total muscle energy production expressed per unit of work (mmol ATP · kg^{-1} w.w. · kJ^{-1}) estimated as the sum of aerobic energy production and anaerobic energy production determined as energy release related to net lactate release, lactate accumulation and utilization of creatine phosphate during the first 20 s and the remaining part of two exhaustive knee-extensor exercise bouts (Ex1 and Ex2) separated by 4 min of rest. *p<0.05: Ex1 significantly different from Ex2.

initial phase that the anaerobic energy production is reduced and the energy turnover per work unit is increased when intense exercise is repeated.

It is unclear what caused a reduction in ATP utilization when intense exercise is repeated. It has been demonstrated that the efficiency of a muscle contraction is increased by prolonged contraction time [12, 13]. However, this does not appear to explain the lower use of energy during the second exercise bout in the studies using one-legged exercise, as there was no indication of a change in the contraction pattern (based on force recordings) from the first to the second exercise bout.

Another possibility is that the fibre type recruitment changed when the exercise was repeated. Certain muscle fibres, particularly fast-twitch (FT) fibres, may not have recovered completely from the first exercise, even after 1 h of rest. As a consequence, more ST fibres could have been involved during the second exercise bout. This may explain the lowered rate of energy utilization, as it has been shown in vitro that ST fibres have a lower energy cost per unit of force [14]. An additional factor may be an elevated efficiency of the FT fibres by the second exercise, as it has been demonstrated that the

ATP turnover in mouse FT muscles decreases as an isometric contraction continues [14].

A third possibility is that ΔG_{ATP} was higher during the second exercise. This may have resulted in a longer movement of the myosin molecule in relation to the actin molecule for each ATP, since it has been suggested that this movement is related to the free energy of ATP. Such changes in movement would have increased the efficiency during the second exercise. A change in ΔG does not appear to be explained by a difference in the level of nucleotides and phosphate, since the concentrations of these compounds were the same when intense exercise was repeated in the one-legged knee-extensor studies [9, 10]. It can, however, not be excluded that there were differences during the exercises, and that the free concentrations of the nucleotides were different. Another possibility is that muscle pH was higher during the second exercise, which may have resulted in higher energy release from ATP. At the end of the exercise bout repeated after 1 h, the muscle lactate was significantly lowered and muscle pH was probably higher, which may explain the higher efficiency in the second exercise bout (fig. 2). In order to examine the effect of pH on energy turnover during intense exercise, an experiment was carried out in which the subjects performed exhaustive knee-extensor exercise on two separate occasions [15]. On one occasion subjects carried out intense intermittent arm exercise prior to exhaustive knee-extensor exercise (Arm exercise – A) and on the other occasion the leg exercise was performed without prior arm exercise (Control – C). The arm exercise resulted in elevated blood lactate concentrations prior to the knee-extensor exercise, which resulted in a lowered lactate release from the leg in A compared to C. Exercise time was 3.46 ± 0.28 and 4.67 ± 0.55 min for A and C, respectively. The energy production expressed per unit of work was not different in the two situations (fig. 4) although muscle pH was lower at the end of exercise in A compared to C (6.65 vs. 6.82; $p < 0.05$). Thus, it appears that muscle pH has little influence on the efficiency of the muscle contractions.

It is clear that further studies are needed to clarify the cause of the reduction in energy turnover, and thus, the increase in mechanical efficiency when intense exercise is repeated.

Oxygen Deficit and Anaerobic Energy Production

Since Krogh and Lindhard [16] in the early part of this century introduced the oxgen deficit concept, the oxygen deficit has frequently been used as a determination of the anaerobic energy production. In one-legged knee-extensor study, the anaerobic energy production determined from changes in

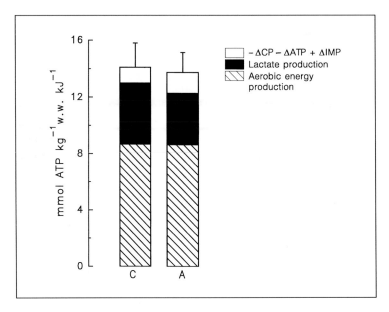

Fig. 4. Total muscle energy production expressed per unit of work (mmol ATP · kg^{-1} w.w. · kJ^{-1}) estimated as the sum of aerobic energy production and anaerobic energy production determined as energy release related to net lactate production and utilization of ATP, creatine phosphate and accumulation of IMP during two exhaustive knee-extensor exercise bouts performed either without (C) or with previous intense intermittent arm exercise (A).

metabolites was close to the anaerobic energy production estimated from the leg O$_2$ deficit, which was determined as the difference between estimated energy demand and total leg oxygen uptake [6]. The close relationship between the two estimations for a single muscle group speaks in favour of using the oxygen deficit also as a measure of the anaerobic energy production during whole-body exercise. However, there appear to be problems with the method when the energy demand is estimated from a linear relationship between oxygen uptake and power output during submaximal exercise.

Firstly, the finding that a group of well-trained runners had a higher oxygen uptake at high submaximal running speeds than the energy demand estimated from a linear relationship between oxygen uptake and lower speeds indicates that the relationship is not linear from low to high submaximal speeds (fig. 5) [17]. Thus, the energy demand during supramaximal intensities may be underestimated when extrapolated from a linear relationship between oxygen uptake and submaximal speeds. This means that the higher the intensity chosen for the supramaximal exercise, the more pronounced the underestimation of the true oxygen deficit.

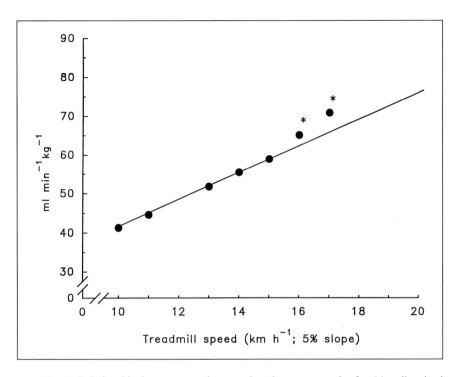

Fig. 5. Relationship between running speed and oxygen uptake for 14 well-trained runners (maximum oxygen uptake: 72.5 ml · min^{-1} · kg^{-1}). The line drawn represents linear regression based on values obtained below 16 km · h^{-1}. *$p < 0.05$: significantly higher than the oxygen uptake estimated from the regression line.

Secondly, it has been observed that the oxygen uptake progressively increases as exercise at high submaximally speeds is continued. This means that the obtained relationship between oxygen uptake and speed is dependent on when the oxygen uptake measurements are performed during the submaximal exercises. Thus, the estimated energy demand during the supramaximal exercise is influenced by the protocol chosen for the submaximal testing.

Thirdly, the anaerobic energy production during submaximal exercise is not taken into account in the calculation of the energy demand during supramaximal exercise. It is well known that blood lactate is elevated during high intensity submaximal exercise, reflecting lactate production in the exercising muscles, and thus representing an anaerobic energy production. The energy production related to lactate production has been estimated to be at least 10% of the aerobic energy production at high intensity submaximal exercise [6].

These findings suggest that the energy demand during supramaximal exercise cannot be estimated from a linear extrapolation from submaximal measurements. The estimation of energy demands during intense exercise are further complicated by the finding that energy turnover per unit of work seems to decrease during intense exercise (fig. 3), suggesting that the energy production during this type of exercise is not constant. It appears that further studies are needed to characterise the energy demand during intense exercise before the oxygen deficit can be used as a measure of the anaerobic energy production.

Conclusion

It appears that the energy turnover per unit of work is lowered, i.e. mechanical efficiency is increased, when intense exercise is repeated. The difference in energy turnover between the first and a subsequent exercise bout is most pronounced in the initial phase of exercise. The oxygen deficit, based on an estimation of the energy demand during intense exercise from a linear relationship between submaximal exercise intensities and oxygen uptake, does not appear to represent the anaerobic energy production during intense exercise.

Acknowledgments

The experiments reported in this article were performed in collaboration with B. Saltin, T. Graham, L. Johansen, B. Kiens, S. Strange, E.A. Richter and B. Quistorff. The studies were supported by grants from Team Danmark, the Danish Natural Science Foundation (11-00820), the Danish National Research Foundation (504–14) and Brandts Legat.

References

1   Wootton SA, Williams C: The influence of recovery duration on repeated maximal sprints; in Knuttgen HG, Vogel JA, Poortmans J (eds): Biochemistry of Exercise. Int Series on Sports Sciences. Human Kinetics Publishers, Champaign, 1983, vol 13, pp 269–273.
2   McCartney N, Spriet LL, Heigenhouser JF, Kowalchuk JM, Sutton, JR, Jones NL: Muscle power and metabolism in maximal intermittent exercise. J Appl Physiol 1986;60:1164–1169.
3   Spriet LL, Lindinger MI, McKelvie S, Heigenhauser GJF, Jones NL: Muscle glycogenolysis and H^+ concentration during maximal intermittent cycling. J Appl Physiol 1989;68:8–13.
4   Gaitanos GC, Williams C, Boobis LH, Brooks S: Human muscle metabolism during intermittent maximal exercise. J Appl Physiol 1993;75:712–719.
5   Bangsbo J: The physiology of soccer with special reference to intense intermittent exercise. Acta Physiol Scand 1994;151 (suppl 619): 1–156.

6   Bangsbo J, Gollnick PD, Graham TE, Juel C, Kiens B, Mizuno M, Saltin B: Anaerobic energy production and O_2 deficit-debt relationship during exhaustive exercise in humans. J Physiol 1990; 422:539–559.

7   Bangsbo J, Gollnick PD, Graham TE, Saltin B: Substrates for muscle glycogen synthesis in recovery from intense exercise in man. J Physiol 1991;434:423–440.

8   Spriet LL, Söderlund K, Bergström M, Hultman E: Anaerobic energy release in skeletal muscle during electrical stimulation in men. J Appl Physiol 1987;62:611–615.

9   Bangsbo J, Graham TE, Kiens B, Saltin B: Elevated muscle glycogen and anaerobic energy production during exhaustive exercise in man. J Physiol 1992;451:205–222.

10 Bangsbo J, Graham TE, Johansen K, Strange S, Christensen C, Saltin B: Elevated muscle acidity and energy production during exhaustive exercise in man. Am J Physiol 1992;263: R891–R899.

11 Sahlin K, Ren JM: Relationship of contraction capacity changes during recovery from a fatiguing contraction. J Appl Physiol 1989;67:648–654.

12 Kushmerick MJ: Patterns in mammalian muscle energetics. J Exp Biol 1985;115:165–167.

13 di Prampero PE, Boutellier U, Marguerat A: Efficiency of work performance and contraction velocity in isotonic tetani of frog sartorius. Pflügers Arch 1988;455–461.

14 Crow MT, Kushmerick MJ: Chemical energetics of slow-and fast-twitch muscles of the mouse. J Gen Physiol 1982;79:147–166.

15 Bangsbo J, Madsen K, Kiens B, Richter EA: Effect of muscle acidity on muscle metabolism and fatigue during intense exercise in man. J Physiol, submitted.

16 Krogh A, Lindhard J: The changes in respiration at the transition from work to rest. J Physiol 1920;53:431–437.

17 Bangsbo J, Petersen A, Michalsik L: Accumulated O_2 deficit during intense exercise and muscle characteristics of elite athletes. Int J Sports Med 1993;14:207–213.

Dr. Jens Bangsbo, The August Krogh Institute, LHF, Universitetsparken 13,
DK–2100 Copenhagen Ø (Denmark)

Marconnet P, Saltin B, Komi P, Poortmans J (eds): Human Muscular Function
during Dynamic Exercise. Med Sport Sci. Basel, Karger, 1996, vol 41, pp 32–43

....
Influence of Body Dimensions, Sex and Training on the Energy Cost of Running

Jean-René Lacour

Physiologie-GIP Exercice, Faculté de Médecine Lyon-Sud, Oullins, France

As early as 1930, Dill et al. [1] reported a difference in excess of 30% in the oxygen demand, as expressed in ml $\cdot$ min^{-1} $\cdot$ kg^{-1}, between subjects running at a standard speed. This demand was further defined as running economy. More recent systematic studies, as reviewed by Daniels [2], evidenced a range of variation of about 20% in running economy, even among well-trained runners. Information relative to the mechanisms reponsible for this interindividual variation is rather scarce. Williams and Cavanagh [3] stated that when studying the mechanical aspects of distance running, no single variable can explain differences in economy between individuals. Kearney and Van Handel [4] reviewed some factors affecting running economy, including age, sex and training status. The purpose of this review is to describe the interplay of body mass with these factors.

The Energy Cost of Running Concept

Comparison between studies is made difficult by the multiple ways of expressing the energy demand of running.

Running economy is considered to be the steady-state oxygen consumption (ml $\cdot$ min^{-1} $\cdot$ kg^{-1}) for a given running speed. This way of expressing the energy demand does not privilege any hypothesis relative to the conversion of oxygen uptake to mechanical work of running. On the other hand, it limits comparison between subjects to those running at the same speed.

The slope of the relation between $\dot{V}O_2$ and running speed would seem to be less dependent on the speed. Kearney and Van Handel [4] reviewed sixteen studies from which this relation could be obtained. The slope values, as expressed in ml · min^{-1} · kg^{-1}/m, ranged from 0.172 to 0.316 in men and from 0.151 to 0.244 in women. In most cases, the y-intercepts of these relationships were negative. Moreover, the authors observed that when comparing the groups, as the capability of the runners improved, the slope of the regression line increased and the y-intercept became more negative. This has been supposed to be a consequence of a possible increase in the oxygen demand as a function of running speed.

Energy Cost of Running

The energy cost of running (C_R), is defined as the energy demand (ml O_2 · kg^{-1} or J · kg^{-1}) per distance unit (m or km). Calculation of this raises some questions.

– The assessment of the energy demand specifically devoted to running implies subtraction of the resting energy consumption. This resting value is different whether it refers to lying quietly or to standing upright on the treadmill before running. The studies of our group here reviewed use the 5 ml · min^{-1} · kg^{-1} value calculated by Medbø et al. [5]. This corresponds to the y-intercept of the regression line calculated from the oxygen uptake measurements obtained on subjects running uphill (6°) at different speeds. This value may be considered as the energy consumption of an individual presenting all the characteristics of a running man, except for running. Whatever the method of assessment, the value obtained does not likely differ from the actual one by more than 1 ml · min^{-1} · kg^{-1}. When related to the oxygen demand corresponding to running at 18–20 km · h^{-1}, i.e. 60–65 ml · min^{-1} · kg^{-1}, such a range of error is of little magnitude.

– Most measurements are conducted at speeds inducing an oxygen consumption lower than $\dot{V}O_{2\,max}$, thus making it possible to use $\dot{V}O_2$ as an indicator of the metabolic demand. C_R may thus be alternatively expressed as oxygen cost (ml O_2 · kg^{-1}), or energy cost (J · kg^{-1}) per distance unit, depending on whether $\dot{V}O_2$ is converted to energy consumption or not. The O_2 energy equivalent depends on the used fuels, as expressed by the respiratory exchange ratio (R). Taking this R value into account may improve the accuracy in C_R assessment. C_R should be measured at running speeds as close as possible to the average velocities sustained during races. However, running at speeds close to maximal aerobic velocity induces an increase in blood lactate concentration, thus raising the question of converting the increase in lactate concentration measured during the running bout into energy expenditure. By taking this energy equivalent (3 ml O_2 · kg^{-1} · mM^{-1}) into account in a group of runners, Di Prampero et al. [6] increased the calculated value of C_R by 2–19%.

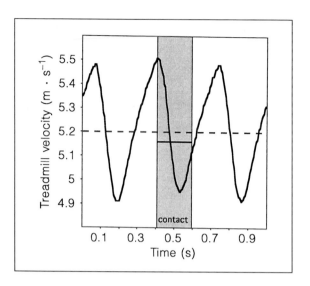

Fig. 1. Evolution of the instantaneous speed of the belt during treadmill running. The contact phase is coincidental with a decrease in speed. This results in an actual running speed slightly lower than the mean belt speed.

Conditions of Measurement

The large range of variation in the energy demand corresponding to the same running speed reported [4] among individuals of similar training status would suggest that the conditions of measurement may constitute a determining factor in this variability. For instance, the possible influence of the expired gas collection apparatus on running technique is not systematically taken into account.

Generally speaking, the question of the validity of any measurement performed during treadmill running may be raised as regards the energy cost of track running. No consistent difference between these two running conditions has ever been demonstrated [7]. Furthermore, treadmill running is biomechanically equivalent to overground running inasmuch as the belt speed is constant [8]. Such a condition is not met as the belt speed is slowed down during each contact phase. This phenomenon also induces an overestimation of the runner's speed when it is calculated from the average speed of the treadmill belt, although the actual running speed is related to the average speed of the belt corresponding to the contact phase (fig. 1). Such an overestimation of the speed results in understimation of C_R. As a matter of fact, treadmill runnning needs training. Brueckner et al. [9] evidenced that at least three bouts of treadmill running have to be performed before C_R stabilizes.

[24] observed that, for a similar training status, women had a slightly higher oxygen cost of running than men. Actually, the differences in m_b were not taken into account in any of these studies. Padilla et al. [29] compared similarly ranking high-level female and male middle-distance runners. The oxygen demands corresponding to the same running speeds were not different. However, women demonstrated a lower C_R/m_b relationship. The lower value of the women's m_b compensated for this lower ratio thus resulting in similar running economies. Sparling and Cureton [30] had already measured identical running economies in male and female recreational runners although the m_b of the women was consistently lower. Helgerud [16] obtained similar results in performance-matched male and female marathon runners. when expressed in $ml \cdot kg^{-0.75} \cdot min^{-1}$, the oxygen demand of women was systematically lower than the men's over running speeds ranging from 160 to 280 m $\cdot$ min^{-1}. However, Daniels and Daniels [31] obtained results which are apparently not in line with the preceding studies. Comparing high-level male and female middle- and long-distance runners they observed that at common test velocities the male runners consumed less oxygen than their female counterparts. This difference, although significant, was less than 1 ml $\cdot$ min$^{-1} \cdot$ kg^{-1}. As the female runners were consistently lighter, their C_R/m_b relationship was lower.

The reason for this difference in the C_R/m_b relationship presumably lies in running mechanics. Williams et al. [12] observed that at the same velocity a group of elite female runners used longer stride lengths and less vertical oscillation (both adjusted to leg length) than their male counterparts. This results in lower mechanical work. On the other hand, Komi and Bosco [32] have pointed out that women were able to utilize a greater portion of the stored elastic energy in counter-movement jumps than men. Bosco et al. [33] have calculated a positive relationship between C_R and the ratio between the mechanical efficiency during jumps performed with and without rebound. Women would thus have a greater capability to spare energy using the stretch-shortening cycle during running. It is worth noting that Bourdin et al. [14], when comparing female basketball players to female runners, observed a lower C_R/m_b relationship in the latter whereas male and female basketball players were not different in this respect. Furthermore, as illustrated by figure 2, male runners and basketball players were not different either. This would lead to suppose that the greater capability to spare energy observed in female runners would result from a greater sensitivity to specific running training.

Women do not demonstrate this lower C_R value during sprint running. Comparison of the blood lactate/velocity relationships obtained during 400-metre races in male and female elite runners [34] showed that women reached the same blood lactate concentrations as men after competitions although their average velocity was 1 m $\cdot$ s^{-1} lower. Thus, as the difference in aerobic capacity is not of great importance in this case, the women's lower performance over this distance would be mostly related to their higher C_R.

Influence of C_R on Performance

As reviewed by Noakes [35] the majority of studies failed to show any significant direct relationship between running economy and athletic performance in middle-distance and endurance running. Actually, performance is related to the combined influence of $\dot{V}O_{2\,max}$, and C_R. The interplay of these two variables has been expressed by the equations constructed by Di Prampero [36]. According to these equations, the maximal speed which can be sustained in aerobic conditions (v_{amax}) is the quotient of the maximal oxygen running demand ($\dot{V}O_{2\,max}-\dot{V}O_{2\,rest}$) by C_R.

$$v_{amax}\,(m \cdot min^{-1}) = \dot{V}O_{2\,max} - \dot{V}O_{2\,rest}\,(ml \cdot kg^{-1} \cdot min^{-1})/C_R\,(ml \cdot kg^{-1} \cdot m^{-1}).$$

The predicted velocity at $\dot{V}O_{2\,max}$ ($v\dot{V}O_{2\,max}$, [2]) is calculated from $\dot{V}O_{2\,max}$, and running economy values measured at several speeds. v_{amax} (or $v\dot{V}O_{2\,max}$) was shown to be correlated with performance over marathon and half-marathon [37], 10,000-metre races [38], and middle-distance races (1,500–5,000 m [34]). These correlations evidence the influence of maximal aerobic power on performances in races lasting more than 3 min. This does not exclude the possible influence of the ability to maintain its C_R with fatigue during running [9]. This ability could account for differences in running performances among subjects demonstrating similar $\dot{V}O_{2\,max}$ and C_R.

The direct influence of either $\dot{V}O_{2\,max}$ and C_R on performance is obscured by the strong correlation relating these two variables. This correlation was first evidenced by Mayhew [39] in male distance runners. It was further evidenced in male middle-distance runners [34] and in female middle-distance runners [29]. This is not a cause-and-effect relationship but likely a consequence of the influence of m_b on both C_R and $\dot{V}O_{2\,max}$ [13]. When expressing C_R as a function of $\dot{V}O_{2\,max}$, each point defined by the coordinates C_R and $\dot{V}O_{2\,max}-5$ corresponds to a v_{amax} value. The iso-v_{amax} lines show that the athletes who exhibit the higher v_{amax} are those who associate a high $\dot{V}O_{2\,max}$ with a middle value of C_R (fig. 4).

Conclusion

C_R directly influences middle-distance and endurance running performances. Comparison of groups differing in age, sex and training reveals that

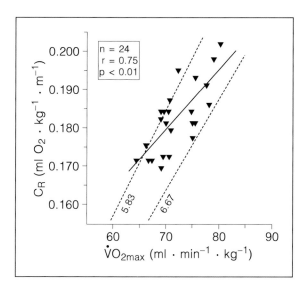

Fig. 4. Relationship between $\dot{V}O_{2\,max}$ and C_R for elite middle-distance runners. Data from Lacour et al. [34].

C_R is not only dependent on body dimensions, but may be sensitive to some factors including training. Advances in the acquisition and analysis of mechanical data and a better understanding of the biomechanics of running would make it possible to disclose factors governing C_R and to develop procedures inducing its improvement.

References

1   Dill DB, Edwards HT, Talbott JH: Studies in muscular activities. VI. Responses of several individuals to a fixed task. J Physiol (Lond) 1930;69:267–305.
2   Daniels JT: A physiologist's view of running economy. Med Sci Sports Exerc 1985;17:332–338.
3   Williams KR, Cavanagh PR: Relationship between distance running mechanics, running economy, and performances. J Appl Physiol 1987;63:1236–1245.
4   Kearney J, Van Handel P: Economy: A physiological perspective. Adv Sports Med Fitness 1989; 2:57–90.
5   Medbø JI, Mohn AC, Tabata I, Bahr R, Vaage O, Sejersted OM: Anaerobic capacity determined by maximal accumulated O_2 deficit. J Appl Physiol 1988;64:50–60.
6   Di Prampero PE, Capelli C, Pagliaro P, Antonutto G, Girardis M, Zamparo P, Soule, RG: Energetics of best performances in middle-distance running. J Appl Physiol 1993;74:2318–2324.
7   Basett DR Jr, Giese MD, Nagle FJ, Ward A, Raab DM, Balke B: Aerobic requirements of overground versus treadmill running. Med Sci Sports Exerc 1985;17:477–481.
8   Van Ingen Schenau GJ: Some fundamental aspects of overground versus treadmill locomotion. Med Sci Sports Exerc 1980;12:257–261.

9   Brueckner JC, Atchou G, Capelli C, Duvallet A, Barrault D, Jousselin E, Rieu M, Di Prampero PE: The energy cost of running increases with the distance covered. Eur J Appl Physiol 1991;62: 385–389.
10   Lacour JR, Bouvat E, Barthélémy JC: Post-competition blood lactate concentrations as indicators of anaerobic energy expenditure. Eur J Appl Physiol 1990;61:172–176.
11   Hautier CA, Wouassi D, Arsac LM, Bitanga E, Thiriet P, Lacour JR: Relationships between post-competition blood lactate and average running velocity over 100-m and 200-m races. Eur J Appl Physiol 1994;68:508–513.
12   Williams KR, Cavanagh PR, Ziff JL: Biomechanical studies of elite female distance runners. Int J Sports Med 1987;8(suppl):107–118.
13   Åstrand PO, Rodahl K: Textbook of Work Physiology. New York, McGraw-Hill, 1986, chapt 9: Body dimensions and muscular exercise.
14   Bourdin M, Pastene J, Germain M, Lacour JR: Influence of training, sex, age and body mass on the energy cost of running. Eur J Appl Physiol 1993;66:439–444.
15   Bergh U, Sjödin B, Forsberg A, Svedenhag J: The relationship between body mass and oxygen uptake during running in humans. Med Sci Sports Exerc 1991;23:205–211.
16   Helgerud J: Maximal oxygen uptake, anaerobic threshold and running economy in women and men with similar performances level in marathons. Eur J Appl Physiol 1994;68:155–161.
17   Davies CTM: Metabolic cost of exercise and physical performance in children with some observations on external loading. Eur J Appl Physiol 1980;45:95–102.
18   Thorstensson A: Effects of moderate external loading on the aerobic demand of submaximal running in men and 10 years-old boys. Eur J Appl Physiol 1986;55:569–574.
19   Cooke CB, McDonagh JN, Nevill AM, Davies CTM: Effects of load on oxygen intake in trained boys and men during treadmill running. J Appl Physiol 1991;71:1237–1244.
20   Åstrand PO: Experimental studies of physical working capacity in relation to sex and age. Copenhagen, Munksgaard, 1952.
21   Krähenbühl GS, Williams TJ: Running economy: Changes with age during childhood and adolescence. Med Sci Sports Exerc 1992;24:462–466.
22   Sjödin B, Svedenhag J: Oxygen uptake during running as related to body mass in circumpubertal boys: A longitudinal study. Eur J Appl Physiol 1992;65:150–157.
23   Daniels J, Oldridge N, Nagle F, White B: Differences and changes in $\dot{V}O_{2\,max}$ among young runners 10 to 18 years of age. Med Sci Sports Exerc 1978;10:200–203.
24   Bransford DR, Howley ET: Oxygen cost of running in trained and untrained men and women. Med Sci Sports 1977;9:41–44.
25   Scrimgeour AG, Noakes TD, Adams B, Myburgh K: The influence of weekly training distance on fractional utilization of maximum aerobic capacity in marathon and ultramarathon runners. Eur J Appl Physiol 1986;55:202–209.
26   Powers S, Dodd S, Deason R, Byrd R, McKnight T: Ventilatory threshold, running economy and distance performance of trained athletes. Res Q Exerc Sport 1983;54:179–182.
27   Svedenhag J, Sjödin B: Body-mass modified running economy and step length in elite male middle- and long-distance runners. Int J Sports Med 1994;15:305–310.
28   Coetzer P, Noakes TD, Sanders B, Lambert MI, Bosch AN, Wiggins T, Dennis SC: Superior fatigue resistance of elite South-African distance runners. J Appl Physiol 1993;75:179–182.
29   Padilla S, Bourdin M, Barthélémy JC, Lacour JR: Physiological correlates of middle-distance running performance. A comparative study between men and women. Eur J Appl Physiol 1992;65:561–566.
30   Sparling PB, Cureton KJ: Biological determinants of the sex difference in 12 min run performance. Med Sci Sports Exerc 1983;15:218–223.
31   Daniels J, Daniels N: Running economy of elite male and elite female runners, Med Sci Sports Exerc 1992;24:483–489.
32   Komi PV, Bosco C: Utilization of stored elastic energy in leg extensor muscles by men and women. Med Sci Sports 1978;10:261–265.
33   Basco C, Montanari G, Ribacchi R, Faina M, Colle R, Dal Monte A, Latteri F, Pastoris F, Benzi G, Cortili G, Saibene F: Relationship between the efficiency of muscular work during jumping and the energetics of running. Eur J Appl Physiol 1987;56:138–143.

34   Lacour JR, Padilla-Magunacelaya S, Barthélémy JC, Dormois D: The energetics of middle-distance running. Eur J Appl Physiol 1990;60:38–43.

35   Noakes TD: Implications of exercise testing for prediction of athletic performance: A contemporary perspective. Med Sci Sports Exerc 1989;20:319–330.

36   Di Prampero PE: The energy cost of human locomotion on land and in water. Int J Sports Med 1986;7:55–72.

37   Di Prampero PE, Atchou G, Brückner JC, Moia C: The energetics of endurance running. Eur J Appl Physiol 1986;55:259–266.

38   Morgan DW, Baldini FD, Martin PE, Kohrt WM: Ten kilometer performance and predicted velocity at $\dot{V}O_{2\,max}$ among well-trained male runners. Med Sci Sports Exerc 1989;21:78–83.

39   Mayhew JL: Oxygen cost and energy expenditure of running in trained runners. Br J Sports Med 1977;11:116–121.

J.R. Lacour, Laboratoire de Physiologie-GIP Exercice, Faculté de Médecine Lyon-Sud,
BP 12, F–69921 Oullins Cédex (France)

Marconnet P, Saltin B, Komi P, Poortmans J (eds): Human Muscular Function
during Dynamic Exercise. Med Sport Sci. Basel, Karger, 1996, vol 41, pp 44–56

....

Mechanical Efficiency of Stretch-Shortening Cycle Exercise

P. V. Komi, H. Kyröläinen

Department of Biology of Physical Activity, University of Jyväskylä, Finland

Conventional classification of muscular function deals with static and dynamic exercises. Static exercise of activated muscle is traditionally referred to as isometric. Force is developed but, as there is no movement, no work is performed. All other muscle actions involve movement and are termed dynamic. The term concentric is traditionally used to identify a shortening action and the term eccentric is used to identify a lengthening action [1].

Isometric and dynamic actions can be assessed at any particular length of the muscle and/or positioning of the related body parts in terms of directly measured force from the muscle or its tendon, force at a particular point on the related body parts, or torque about the axis of rotation. A dynamic action must be further described in terms of directionality (shortening or lengthening) and the velocity of muscle length change or body part movement.

Stretch-Shortening Cycle of Muscle Function

Muscular exercises seldom involve pure forms of isolated isometric, concentric or eccentric actions. This is because the body segments are periodically subjected to impact forces, as in running or jumping, or because some external force such as gravity lengthens the muscle. In these phases, the muscles are acting eccentrically, and concentric action follows. By definition of eccentric action, the muscles must be active during the stretching phase. The combination of eccentric and concentric actions forms a natural type of muscle function called a stretch-shortening cycle (SSC) [2, 3].

The purpose of SSC is to make the final action (concentric phase) more powerful than that resulting from the concentric action alone. Since Cavagna

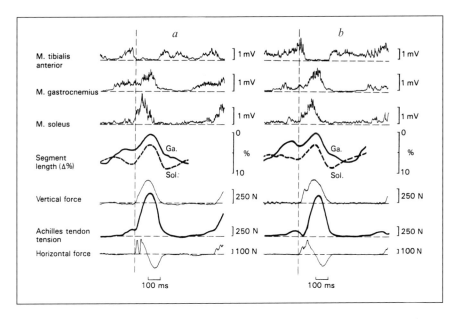

Fig. 1. A representative record of the ATF and segmental length changes of the gastro-cnemius (Ga) and soleus (Sol) muscles together with Fz and Fy ground reaction forces and selected EMG activities when the subject was running along a long force platform. The vertical line indicates the beginning of the ground contact as well as of the SSC of the muscles. The upward and downward deflections of the segmental length changes signify, respectively, stretching (eccentric) and shortening (concentric) phases of the cycle. *a* Ball running. *b* Heel running. Data from Komi [6].

et al. [4] introduced the basic mechanisms of work enhancement when an isolated muscle was subjected to active stretch (eccentric action) prior to its shortening (concentric action), considerable scientific work has been devoted to explaining the detailed mechanisms of force and power potentiation in SSC [5].

Direct in vivo Achilles tendon force (ATF) measurements can be used to demonstrate SSC during normal locomotion [7]. Figure 1 presents typical results of SSC for the soleus and gastrocnemius muscles separately in running. Several important features are to be noted. First, the changes in muscle-tendon length are very small during the stretching phase. This suggests that the conditions favour the potential utilization of short-range stiffness in the muscle [8]. Second, the segmental length changes in these two muscles take place in phase in both the lengthening and shortening parts of the SSC. This is typical for running and jumping; it has considerable importance because

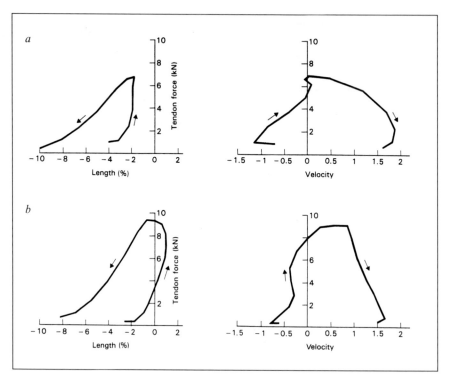

Fig. 2. Instantaneous force-length and force-velocity curves of the gastrocnemius muscle for SSC when the subject ran at two different velocities. The upward deflection signifies stretching (eccentric action) and the downward deflection shortening (concentric action) of the muscle. Data from Komi [6]. *a* 9.02 m · s^{-1}. *b* 5.78 m · s^{-1}.

the transducer measures forces of the common tendon for the two muscles. The situation is not so simple in other activities, such as bicycling [9] where the length changes are more out of phase in these two muscles. The third important feature of the example in figure 1 is that the form of the ATF curve, resembles that of a bouncing ball.

The force-length and force-velocity curves can then be computed on the basis of the curves, as presented in figure 1. It must be emphasized that in this analysis, the force values represent the two muscles simultaneously, because AT is common to both of them. Figure 2 presents such an analysis during the contact phase in running. The force-length curve demonstrates a very sharp increase in force during the stretching phase, which is characterized by a small change in length. The right side of the figure shows the force-velocity comparison demonstrating high potentiation during the stretching phase (concentric action). The muscle length estimates that were used have shown that running and jumping are not the only activities where SSC can be identified. Evidence [9, 10] has demonstrated that the gastrocnemius and soleus muscles also function in bicycling in SSC, although the stretching phases are not as apparent as in running or jumping.

The major conclusion from the various studies, both human and animal, is that SSC muscle action produces muscle outputs which can be very different from the conditions of isolated preparations, where activation levels are held constant and storage of strain energy is limited. Furthermore, it can be stated that, if the mechanical outputs of the muscle are enhanced in SSC action, the logical consequence should be that the work efficiency is enhanced as well.

Mechanical Efficiency

Mechanical efficiency (ME) has been studied for almost a century and the textbooks of physiology have until recently referred to mechanical efficiency (ME) varying between 20 and 25%. Experiments conducted primarily during the last two decades have shed some doubts on such a relatively low level of ME which varied only slightly. It is now known that the different forms of muscle action have a different ME and that the velocity of shortening and stretching influences its value [11–13]. In addition, SSC alone may introduce very different loading conditions and subsequently different ME.

In our laboratory, we have performed several experiments with a special sledge apparatus (fig. 3), which makes it possible to study the isolated forms of concentric and eccentric exercises as well as SSC exercise. The results have indicated that ME in isolated concentric exercises is not constant but varies between 14 and 18% being lower with higher shortening velocities. In pure eccentric exercise, ME increases as a function of stretch velocity and can reach values over 60% [13].

Methodological Consideration to Estimate Mechanical Efficiency in Stretch-Shortening Cycle

During SSC exercise, the definition of ME follows the traditional computation in which the determinants of ME, external work and energy expenditure, must be estimated as accurately as possible. The methods employed have varied slightly depending on the exercise type and availability of equipment. In cycling, for example, the external work has generally been calculated by multiplying the load by the frequency [15]. In walking and running, film analysis has been employed in most cases to define mechanical work as a sum of internal and external work [16, 17]. In jumping, video analysis has been used simultaneously

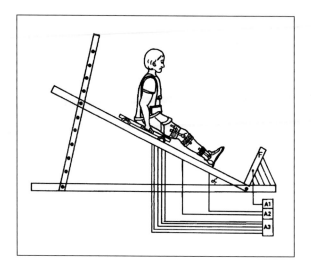

Fig. 3. Diagram of the experimental system used for the study of ME of either isolated eccentric and concentric exercise and their combination SSC. The subject is tightly fixed with belts on to the sledge having an inclination (α) of 22.5°. F and A1 = Forceplate and its amplifer, A2 = amplifiers of the electrical goniometers for the knee and for the ankle; A3 = electromyographic amplifiers. Modified from Kaneko et al. [12].

with the measurements of ground reaction forces [18]. Recently, video analysis and force measurements have also been combined in rowing [19] to calculate the total mechanical work done using dynamic methods [20, 21].

Energy expenditure has usually been measured indirectly from the expired air. CO_2 and O_2 concentrations can be assessed either by a manually operated chemical analyser or by more sophisticated automatic systems. Based on these two determinants, ME is then a proportion of the amount of the work done for the energy expended. For determining ME in a more controlled condition of SSC exercise a special sledge apparatus was again employed and developed further [13, 22]. SSC performance (sledge jump) starts when the assistants drop the subject from a predetermined dropping height causing differences in the stretch velocity of the leg extensor muscles. The initial braking (eccentric) phase follows immediately the push-off (concentric) phase of a predetermined intensity. The assistants select the required dropping height, and inform the subject of the height to which the sledge has been risen to.

A force platform placed perpendicularly to the sliding surface is used to measure the reaction forces as well as the beginning and the end of the contact. The distance the sledge moved and its velocity are measured by an optical encoder. Thereafter, the external work is calculated by the integral of the function F(x) between the limit p_1 and p_2 as follows:

$$W_{tot} = \int_{p_1}^{p_2} F(x)dx, \tag{1}$$

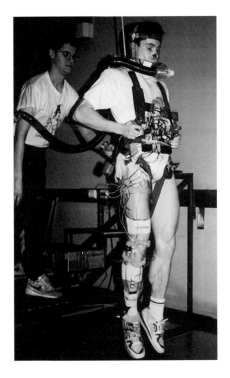

Fig. 4. A subject performing drop jump exercises for estimation of ME. Data from Kyröläinen and Komi [22].

where F = the reaction force, x = the displacement of the sledge, p_1 = the position of the sledge in the beginning of the contact, p_2 = the position of the sledge in the end of the contact with the force plate.

For inducing a more reactive jumping performance as compared to the sledge jumps, drop jump exercises can also be utilised. In these submaximal drop jumps (fig. 4), instructions for the subjects are to maximally resist the downward movement during the braking phase, bend the knees minimally, and perform a submaximal push-off phase during the take-off. The subjects perform e.g. 60 muscle actions which last a total of 3 min. In this case, the frequency is once every 3 s and is controlled by an audiosignal. When the subject leaves the ground contact, two assistants use a rope attached to the subject's vest and pull him up to the same energy level by a special pulley system for the next drop. The third assistant takes care of the subject's balance during this phase. For more details, the reader is referred to Kyröläinen and Komi [22].

Simultaneously with the force recordings, angular displacements of the knee and ankle joints are measured by electrogoniometers, and electromyographic (EMG) activity of leg extensor muscles is recorded telemetrically with surface electrodes. The expired gases are analysed by measuring pulmonary oxygen uptake, the volume of the air, and its concentrations of O_2 and CO_2 by using a semi-automatic gas analyser.

After all these recordings, the net energy expenditure (ΔE) is determined by the oxygen consumption. The oxygen uptake (VO_2) and respiratory exchange ratio ($R = VCO_2 \cdot VO_2^{-1}$)

for every 30 s. Measurements must be made before exercise (rest VO_2), during exercise and during the recovery period until the VO_2 returns to the resting level. The rest VO_2 is subtracted from the total consumption of the oxygen. To calculate the energy expenditure, an energy equivalent of 20,180 J/l of oxygen is applied, when R is 0.82. The change of 0.01 in R-value caused a change of 42 J in energy expenditure. Thereafter, each R-value of every 30 s is multiplied by the respective value of O_2 ($1 \cdot min^{-1}$) to obtain ΔE. Its mean value (work + recovery) is then utilized in further calculations.

Finally, the ME of the total work (W_{tot}) is calculated as follows:

$$ME = \frac{W_{tot}}{\Delta E} \cdot 100\%. \tag{2}$$

Major Findings

Earlier studies have demonstrated that a short and rapid stretch with a short coupling time and a high force at the end of prestretch creates a good precondition for utilizing tendomuscular elasticity. However, the force attained at the end of the stretching period depends on the amplitude and the velocity of the stretch [23]. During jumping with higher angular velocities of the knee joint ME increases [18]. This is also the case when the amplitude of the knee bending in the braking phase decreases [13]. In addition, it has been shown that the net ME of positive work increases with increased prestretch intensity [13, 14]. Figure 5 demonstrates that total ME increased also individually within certain limits, with increased stretching velocity of the leg extensor muscles reaching values in the range of 42.8–69.0% with faster stretches [22]. This phenomenon seems to be related to the occurrence of EMG potentiation in the higher prestretch intensity during the eccentric phase of SSC exercise [14]. In other words, muscle stiffness may increase, with certain incremental limits of prestretch intensity causing better utilization of tendomuscular elasticity and, finally, increase in ME. It seems, however, that when the tendomuscular stretch is excessive, ME may start to plateau or even decrease.

The present method has also been utilised to study training adaptation of ME [24]. Power type strength training improved ME (fig. 6); this was associated with changes in muscle activity patterns of the leg extensor muscles. After training, the subjects preactivated their muscles earlier before the impact. During the braking phase of the take-off, clear disappearance of segmentation of the EMG curves was observed. This could imply modification of muscle stiffness and recoil characteristics of the tendomuscular complex. At the same time, demands of energy expenditure could decrease with subsequent increase of ME.

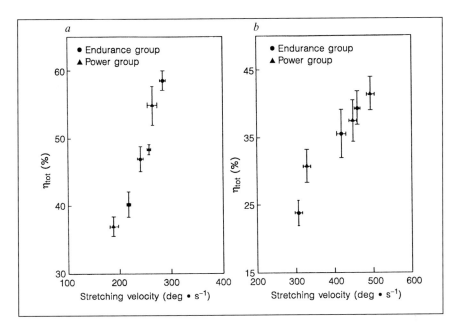

Fig. 5. The mean (±SE) values of the total mechanical efficiency related to the respective values of the stretching velocity determined indirectly by the angular velocity of the knee joint during the sledge jumps (*a*) and during the drop jumps (*b*). Data from Kyröläinen and Komi [22].

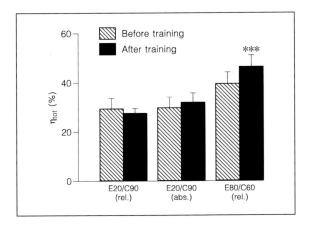

Fig. 6. Mean (±SD) values of the total mechanical efficiency of SSC exercises before power-type strength training and after 16 weeks of training. The two dropping heights on the sledge were 20 cm (E20) and 80 cm (E80), while the intensity of the positive work was 60% (C60) or 90% (C90) of the single maximal concentric exercises. ***p < 0.001. Data from Kyröläinen et al. [24].

Methodological Problems

There exist many problems, encountered by any method of estimating ME and, especially, its determinant of mechnical work. How to take into account all distributions of potential (elastic and gravitational) and kinetic (linear and rotational) energy sources [19] or how to determine internal and external work [17]? Martin et al. [25] demonstrated that the total mechanical work (external work) provided a better explanation for the aerobic demands in locomotion than the segment-based model (external + internal work). On the other hand, 'it is shown that external and mechanical work depend on each other and their sum is not equal to the mechanical energy expenditure which occurs during movement of the body' [21]. Therefore, Aleshinsky [20] developed a dynamic method to determine total mechanical work. It is based on calculations of the sum of work done around each joint. However, in spite of many studies in the field of ME, the contributions of elastic energy, co-activation of agonist and antagonist muscles, and the multijoint action of some muscles are still unclear.

EMG recordings have clarified some of the problems involved in estimations of ME. In several studies, a constant value of -1.2 (120%) [11] has been used as ME value of the eccentric part of the SSC exercise [18, 26]. The use of the sledge apparatus in studying ME of the positive work in SSC exercise was thought to be an improvement in this respect. Indeed, this method demonstrated quite conclusively that ME in pure eccentric exercise is a function of stretch velocity. Consequently no constant value can be given to the ME of eccentric exercise. The calculation of positive work of ME in SSC exercise was based on the assumption that the eccentric phase of the SSC condition was the same as in the pure eccentric condition with the same dropping height of the sledge. The EMG values, however, demonstrate that this was not the case (fig. 7) [13]. In fact, in the isolated condition, the EMGs were, much lower than in a comparable eccentric phase of SSC exercise. Thus, despite the apparently same mechanical work, the energy expenditures must have been different. Higher EMG values would imply higher energy expenditure when two types of eccentric phases, which have the same mechanical work, are compared with each other. This naturally introduces errors in the final calculations of ME in the positive work phase in SSC and the final result will probably be an overestimation [14].

The third unsolved problem is associated with the calculation of energy expenditure. When the work intensity is low, on an aerobic level, the values of oxygen uptake and respiratory ratio give enough information for determining energy expenditure. However, if the subjects are working on an anaerobic level, their true energy cost can be underestimated and, therefore, their ME

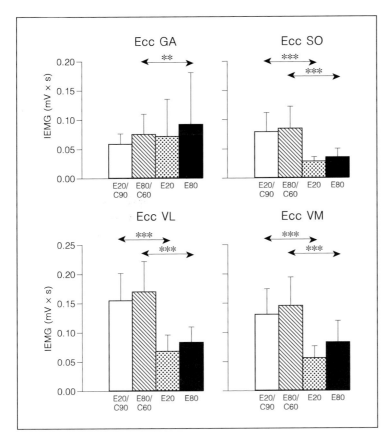

Fig. 7. Integrated EMG (IEMG) (mean ± SD) during sledge exercises from the gastrocnemius (GA), soleus (SO), vastus lateralis (VL) and vastus medialis (VM) muscles from the eccentric (Ecc) phase of the SSC exercises (E20/C90 and E80/C60) and during the pure eccentric exercises (E20 and E80). **p < 0.01, ***p < 0.001. C60 and C80 represent concentric muscle actions of 60% and 90% of maximum, respectively. E20 and E80 are the dropping heights of 20 cm and 80 cm and characterize the respective eccentric exercises. Data from Kyröläinen et al. [14].

values become overestimated. The studies of Ribeiro et al. [27] and Di Prampero et al. [28] have suggested that when blood lactate is higher than at rest, and constant in time, it necessarily follows that both lactate production and its removal have increased by the same amount. Thus the extra lactate produced in some muscles is oxidised in other muscles and organs. The recent studies of Bangsbo et al. [29] and Di Prampero et al. [30] have estimated the value of oxygen debt (lactate production) as an energy yield. In spite of that, more studies are needed to estimate the contribution of lactate and other possible substrates as an energy yield during anaerobic work.

Mechanical Efficiency in Running

As has already been emphasized in this paper, running is a very typical form of SSC exercise for the lower extensor muscles. Several cross-sectional studies have been published on running economy and/or its ME. Recently, a new method has been developed for studying mechanical work during running [31]. The external work of subjects was determined by a kinematic arm, which is a device for three-dimensional recording of human movement. It consists of four rigid bars linked together by three joints equipped with optical transducers. One end of the kinematic arm is connected to a fixed reference point while the other end is fixed to the back of the subject, near the centre of gravity of the whole body, and can move freely in the three spatial directions. For more details of this method, see Belli et al. [31] and Kyröläinen et al. [32].

This method has been used in the study where the subjects ran 5 min at the two predetermined constant speeds of $2.50 \text{ m} \cdot \text{s}^{-1}$ and $3.25 \text{ m} \cdot \text{s}^{-1}$ on the treadmill and on the track. The velocity of the treadmill was measured by means of an optical encoder. During running on the track, the running velocity and the mechanical work were measured by the same method as on the treadmill. The measuring equipment was placed in an electric car, which was driven on the side of the subject. The running speed of the subject was paced by the driver of the car. He drove around the 200-metre-long track at the predetermined constant speed by following the pointer of a speedometer, which was connected to the optical encoder. The air expired for 1 min was collected into the Douglas bag during the period of the steady-state oxygen uptake (from 4 to 5 min or in some cases from 3 to 4 min). The volume of air in the Douglas bag was determined by a gasometer, and its concentrations of O_2 and CO_2 by the same gas analyser as in the treadmill running.

The results demonstrated that, as was the case for the sledge and jumping exercises, ME in running was also relatively high (from 36.3 to 59.6%, individually) during the two measured speeds and they differed only slightly between track and treadmill running. Thus the two methods employed to calculate external mechanical work (sledge method vs. kinematic arm) behaved in the same way with regard to the values of ME in the total SSC cycle. It is true that the obtained ME values are suprisingly high but we believe that only part of the problem may be explained by possible errors in calculating both the external work and energy expenditure. Thus it seems that human locomotion with regard to the SSC type exercise is relatively efficient.

References

1　Knuttgen HG, Komi PV: Basic definitions for exercise; in Komi PV (ed): Strength and Power in Sport. Blackwell Scientific Publications, Oxford, 1992, pp 3–6.

2　Norman RW, Komi PV: Electromyographic in skeletal muscle under normal movement conditions. Acta Physiol Scand 1979;106:241–248.

3　Komi PV: Physiology and biomechanical correlates of muscle function: Effects of muscle structure and stretch-shortening cycle on force and speed; in Terjung RH (ed): Exercise and Sport Sciences Reviews, Lexington, DC Health, 1984, vol 12, pp 81–123.

4　Cavagna GA, Saibene FP, Margaria R: Effect of negative work on the amount of positive work performed by an isolated muscle. J Appl Physiol 1965;20:157–158.

5　Huijing PA: Elastic potential of muscle; in Komi PV (ed): Strength and Power in Sport. Blackwell Scientific Publications, Oxford, 1992, pp 151–168.

6　Komi PV: Stretch-shortening cycle; in Komi PV (ed): Strength and Power in Sport. Blackwell Scientific Publications, Oxford, 1992, pp 169–179.

7　Komi PV: Relevance of in vivo force measurements to human biomechanics. J Biomech 1990; 23(suppl 1):23–24.

8　Rack PM, Westbury DR: The short range stiffness of active mammalian muscle and its effect on mechanical properties. J Physiol (Lond) 1974;240:331–350.

9　Gregor RJ, Komi PV, Browing RL, Järvinen M: A comparison of the triceps surae and residual muscle moments at the ankle during cycling. Int J Sports Med 1991;8(suppl):287–297.

10　Gregor RJ, Komi PV, Järvinen M: Achilles tendon forces during cycling. Int J Sports Med 1967; 8(suppl):9–14.

11　Margaria R: Positive and negative work performance and their efficiences in human locomotion. Int Z Angew Physiol Einschl Arbeitsphysiol 1968;25:339–351.

12　Kaneko M, Komi, PV, Aura O: Mechanical efficiency of concentric and eccentric excercises performed with medium to fast contraction rates. Scand J Sport Sci 1984;1:15–20.

13　Aura O, Komi PV: Effects of prestretch intensity on mechanical efficiency of positive work and on elastic behavior of skeletal muscle in stretch-shortening cycle exercise. Int J Sports Med 1986;7: 137–143.

14　Kyröläinen H, Komi PV, Oksanen P, Häkkinen K, Cheng S, Kim DH: Mechanical efficiency of locomotion in females during different kinds of muscle action. Eur J Appl Physiol 1990;61: 446–452.

15　Abbot BC, Aubert XM: The force exerted by active striated muscle during and after change of length. J Physiol (Lond) 1952;117:77–86.

16　Cavagna GA, Kaneko M: Mechanical work and efficiency in level walking and running. J Physiol (Lond) 1977;268:467–481.

17　Winter DA: A new definition of mechanical work done in human movement. J Appl Physiol 1979; 46:79–83.

18　Bosco C, Ito A, Komi PV, Luhtanen P, Rahkila P, Rusko H, Viitasalo JT: Neuromuscular function and mechanical efficiency of human leg extensor muscles during jumping exercises. Acta Physiol Scand 1982;114:543–550.

19　Smith R, Milburn P: A comparison of two methods of assessing mechanical energy expenditure during maximal ergometer rowing; in Bouisset S, Métral S, Monod H (eds): Proceedings of Biomechanics XIV. Paris, pp 1264–1265.

20　Aleshinsky SY: An energy 'source' and 'fractions' approach to the mechanical energy expenditure problem I. Basic concepts, description of the model, analysis of a one-link system movement. J Biomech 1986;19:287–293.

21　Aleshinsky SY: An energy 'sources' and 'fractions' approach to the mechanical energy expenditure problem. II. Movement of the multi-link chain model. J Biomech 1986;19:295–300.

22　Kyröläinen H, Komi PV: Differences in mechanical efficiency between power- and endurance-trained athletes while jumping. Eur J Appl Physiol 1995;70:36–44.

23　Cavagna GA, Dusman B, Margaria R: Positive work done by a previously stretched muscle. J Appl Physiol 1968;24:21–32.

---

24 Kyröläinen H, Komi PV, Kim DH: Effects of power training on neuromuscular performance and mechanical efficiency. Scand J Med Sci Sports 1991;1:78–87.
25 Martin PE, Heise GD, Morgan DW: Interrelationships between mechanical power, energy transfers, and walking and running economy. Med Sci Sports Exerc 1993;25:508–515.
26 Ito A, Komi PV, Sjödin B, Bosco C, Karlsson J: Mechanical efficiency of positive work in running at different speeds. Med Sci Sports Exerc. 1983;15:299–308.
27 Ribeiro JP, Hughes V, Fielding RA, Holden W, Evans W, Knuttgen HG: Metabolic and ventilatory responses to steady state excrcise relative to lactate thresholds. Eur J Appl Phys 1986;55:215–221.
28 Di Prampero PE: The anaerobic threshold concept: A critical evaluation. Adv Cardiol 1986;35: 24–34.
29 Bangsbo J, Gollnick PD, Graham TE, Juel C, Kiens B, Mizuno M, Saltin B: Anaerobic energy production and O_2 deficit-debt relationship during exhaustive exercise in humans. J Physiol (Lond) 1990;422:539–559.
30 Di Prampero PE, Capelli C, Pagliaro P, Antonutto G, Girardis M, Zampero P, Soule RG: Energetics of best performances in middle-distance running. J Appl Physiol 1993;74:2318–2324.
31 Belli A, Rey S, Bonnefoy R, Lacour JR: A simple device for kinematic measurements of human movement. Ergonomics 1993;35:177–186.
32 Kyröläinen H, Komi PV, Belli A: Mechanical efficiency in athletes during running. Scand J Med Sci Sports 1995;5:200–208.

Prof. P.V. Komi, Department of Biology of Physical Activity, University of Jyväskylä, Seminaarinkatu 15, FIN–40100 Jyväskylä (Finland)

Marconnet P, Saltin B, Komi P, Poortmans J (eds): Human Muscular Function
during Dynamic Exercise. Med Sport Sci. Basel, Karger, 1996, vol 41, pp 57–70

....

Measurement of Mechanical Factors of Running Efficiency

Alain Belli

Laboratoire de Physiologie-GIP Exercice, Faculté de Médecine Lyon-Sud,
Oullins, France

In physical activities the efficiency is defined by the ratio of the mechanical
energy produced (EP) by the muscles to the metabolic energy consumption
(EC) [1]. Therefore, in order to calculate the efficiency of any physical activity,
one must be able to define and measure both the numerator and the denomin-
ator, respectively EP and EC, of the efficiency equation. However, the application of such a simple concept to running activity is not obvious.

Measurement of Metabolic Energy Consumption

Historically, precise measurements of EC were obtained before EP measurements. As reviewed by Margaria [2], one century ago, many authors were
already able to estimate the energy consumption of locomotion from CO_2
production. It is now well established that in aerobic conditions, metabolic
energy consumption can be exactly calculated from both the measurement of
oxygen uptake ($\dot{V}O_2$) and CO_2 production ($\dot{V}CO_2$). For instance, for exercise
performed at 50% of the maximal oxygen uptake ($\dot{V}O_{2\,max}$), the respiratory
exchange ratio ($\dot{V}CO_2 \times \dot{V}O_2^{-1}$) is about 0.85 and 1 litre of O_2 consumed is
equivalent to 20,450 J energy consumption [3].

As a consequence of accurate EC measurement possibilities, a first
approach of the 'efficiency' of running was to examine the oxygen uptake of
runners during submaximal bouts. It has been found that, in association with
the subject's $\dot{V}O_{2\,max}$, the energy cost of running (C_R), defined as the oxygen
consumption per kilogram body weight and per metre, is an important factor
of running performance [4]. As reviewed by Lacour [5] in this issue a range

of variation of about 20% in C_R could be measured among well-trained athletes. Although the interindividual variations of C_R have been extensively studied [6], and could provide significant insights in the energetics of running [7], it is worth noting that it does not give any information on the mechanics of running and thus cannot be directly interpreted as differences in mechanical efficiency.

Calculation of Mechanical Energy Production

Since Newton established the equations of classic mechanics, it is possible to precisely determine the mechanical energy changes of moving masses. Therefore it should be theoretically possible to compute EP from kinematic and kinetic measurements during human movement. However, calculation of the exact energy production of muscles from kinetic and kinematic measurement only is not so obvious. As a consequence, three different methods of calculation of EP were successively proposed by researchers.

The first method, proposed by Fenn [8] in 1930, is based on kinematic measurements of the centre of mass of the body (CM). The potential and kinetic energies of CM are computed from the measurement of respectively the vertical displacement and the horizontal velocity changes of CM. Because potential and kinetic CM energies are in phase during running [9], their summation gives the total mechanical energy of CM (EP_{CM}). The rotational kinetic energy, due to the rotation of the limbs relatively to CM, could additionally be measured and provide the 'internal energy' while the sum of potential and translational kinetic energy was mentioned to be 'external energy' [8, 9].

The second method, detailed by Winter [10] in 1979, is based on kinematic measurements of body segments. The total mechanical energy level of the body is the sum of the potential and kinetic energies of each segment (EP_{SEG}). Because potential and kinetic energy changes of segments are not in phase, transfers of energy within an between segments should be taken into consideration in the computation of the total mechanical energy. Depending on the authors, energy transfer within and/or between segments was arbitrarily taken or not into account and these different models of computation could lead to very different total energy computations [11].

In 1986, Aleshinsky [12–14] validated a third method based on both kinematic and kinetic measurements [15]. In this method the mechanical energy is computed from segment dynamics and associated net joint forces and moments (EP_{DYN}). The same author also demonstrated that the sum of external and internal works does not give the total mechanical work [13] and that all the computation methods based on only kinematic measurement of body segments 'do not correspond to the essence phenomena underlying muscular activity' [14]. As a consequence, only the method based on both kinematic and kinetic measurements should provide the best theoretical way to compute the mechanical energy expenditure of the whole body.

However, because the human musculoskeletal system is highly redundant, the same movement pattern can be generated by different combinations of forces of the muscles possibly involved in the movement. For instance, energy could (or not) be transferred by two joint muscles [16]. Although optimisation techniques have been developed [17, 18], it is still not possible to determine the exact contribution of all muscles during multijoint movements from external measurement only. Nevertheless, precise mechanical computations could be performed for single-joint movements [19] and promising invasive methods [20] could probably be applied in future for multijoint calculations.

The Paradox of Mechanical Work of Running

In addition to the problem encountered in determining the exact muscle mechanical work, it is worth noting that, whatever the method of calculation of the mechanical work, the applications of Newton's laws to running mechanics lead us to an apparent paradox. Considering the entire body as an isolated mechanical system and assuming that the work due to the friction effects is negligible [21], the mechanical energy level of the system is not changed in a cyclic motion movement like running. In fact, exactly the same amounts of negative and positive work are absorbed and produced, respectively, and thus the total resulting mechanical work is nil. The concomitant measurement of energy expenditure seems then to be paradoxical.

The answer to that paradox is that muscles are not recuperative sources, in other words, muscles are not able to store mechanical energy during negative phases and to re-use it during positive phases. This phenomenon has been empirically taken into account by separating the phases of positive and negative energy changes during movement. Depending on the authors, EP was calculated only from positive energy changes [9] or from the addition of absolute values of both negative and positive energy changes [10, 11]. In the latter case the EP values would be double the EP values calculated only from positive energy changes.

In fact, it has been shown that muscles are partly recuperative when they are actively stretched immediately before shortening [22–24]. This phenomenon, called stretch-shortening cycle and detailed by Komi and Kyröläinen [25] in this issue, occurs during running [9, 24, 26]. Unfortunately, in isolated muscle preparations [23, 27] as well as in human movement [20, 28], the amount of energy which could be re-used in stretch-shortening cycle depends on external force-velocity conditions and on functional differences between muscles and subjects [29, 30]. Therefore it seems very difficult to calculate the influence of stretch-shortening cycle in the mechanical energy production of all the muscles involved in a complex human movement.

Measurement of Running Efficiency

The enormous range of running efficiency values found in the literature (from 31% up to 197%) [31] reflects the differences in computation methods used by researchers to calculate EP [32].

It could be argued that the differences observed in efficiency values as well as the lack of relationship between EC and EP could also be due to the accuracy of the measurement methods. The coefficient of variation during test-retest EC measurements is about 3% including both biological and methodological variations [3]. The differences observed for external mechanical work ranged from 1.4% to 12.3%, depending on the measurement method [33, 34]. Therefore, although the EC and EP measurement errors are consistent, they could probably explain only a minor part of the discrepancy in efficiency values previously found in the literature.

In fact, as was previously discussed, because of redundancy and recuperative possibilities of the musculoskeletal system, there is no kinematic and/or kinetic measurement method giving the exact EP during running. Such methodological difficulties prevent us from calculating the exact efficiency value of running. However, it would be of interest to determine whether one of the EP computation methods, if there are any, could provide a better understanding of the mechanical factors influencing the efficiency of running. An answer to that question could be found by examining the possible relationships between inter-individual C_R variations and running mechanics [35] with special reference to EP computations.

As reviewed by Morgan et al. [36], it is very difficult to find biomechanical variables in the literature consistently related to the interindividual C_R differences in subjects compared at the same running velocity. For instance, Williams and Cavanagh [35] measured several biomechanical parameters in 31 runners, including three-dimensional kinematic parameters, ground reaction forces and mechanical power computed from kinematic measurements of body segments. It appeared that none of these biomechanical parameters could clearly explain the interindividual differences in C_R. However, as C_R is a global index of energy consumption, significant relationship between EP and C_R could be expected. In a recent study. Martin et al. [37] answered that point negatively.

Whatever the method of computation (EP_{CM}, EP_{SEG} or EP_{DYN}), the interindividual differences in EP calculated in 30 subjects were not significantly related to the corresponding C_R differences. Surprisingly, the best tendency ($p < 0.1$, $r = 0.40$) was obtained with EP_{CM}, which is the simplest method to calculate mechanical energy. Therefore it is concluded that the mechanical parameters responsible for C_R differences could not be identified in the previously described measurements.

The Kinematic Arm Method

The methods usually applied for kinematic measurements in running are film or video analysis. The recordings are later digitised for computation of the displacement and the velocity of body segments. Knowing the mass and the inertia of the segments, it is possible to compute EP_{CM} and EP_{SEG}. Combined with force platform measurements, these data provide EP_{DYN}. These methods have been extensively described and applied and it is not the purpose of this article to further discuss them. However, because they are expensive and difficult to handle, the number of successive steps measured and analysed is limited. The consequences of this limitation on the accuracy of kinematic calculations have been studied by means of a new measurement method.

In order to be able to measure mechanical parameters in a large number of steps and in many subjects, kinematic arm (KA) allowing fast and easy measurement of the body displacements in the three spatial dimensions has been designed. The KA consists of four light, rigid bars linked together by three mono-axial joints. A special orientation of the axis of the joints allows the measuring end of the KA to move freely in the three spatial directions while the other end is connected to a reference point. At each joint an optical transducer interfaced to a PC computer measures the joint angles. Knowing the bar length and the joint angles, an appropriate trigonometric equation could be applied by the computer to calculate the instantaneous position of the moving end relative to the reference end [33]. In order to apply the KA method to running, the measuring end of the KA is linked to the subject by means of a belt fastened around his waist (fig. 1). It has been shown that in running the accuracy of measurements obtained with the KA is comparable to or better than the accuracy of the measurements obtained with video or film analysis [33, 34].

The kinematic arm was applied to measure selected mechanical parameters (vertical body oscillation and step time) of 17 subjects during treadmill running [38]. They ran successively at 60, 80, 100 and 140% of their maximal aerobic velocity. As much as 6,116 steps were measured and analysed. The step time variability ranged from 1.7 to 15.6% while the vertical oscillation

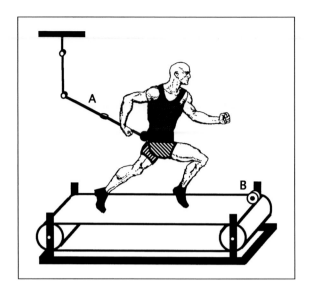

Fig. 1. Schematic view of KA measurement during running. A and B are the KA and the belt displacement transducer, respectively. Data from Belli et al. [38].

variability ranged from 5.5 to 37.3%. For submaximal velocity levels, the variabilities were independent of velocity whereas differences between subjects were significant ($p < 0.01$). Furthermore, the vertical oscillation variability was roughly ($r^2 = 0.24$) but significantly linked ($p < 0.05$) to the intra-individual C_R differences.

An important methodological consequence of step variability is that, in order to be accurate, measurement of mechanical parameters during running must be performed and averaged on a large amount of steps. For instance, the error done on vertical body oscillation, characterised by a variability of 32%, could be as high as 288% if this parameter were measured on only two steps [38]! It was then suggested that the lack of correlation observed between metabolic energy consumption and mechanical energy production in previous studies could be due not only to measurement accuracy or to the impossibility to compute the exact muscle work, but to the low number of steps measured.

Relationship between Energy Production and Energy Cost of Running

The kinematic arm method has been recently applied by Bourdin et al. [39, 40] to mechanical energy computations during treadmill running. Ten trained male runners were asked to perform running bouts on treadmill at

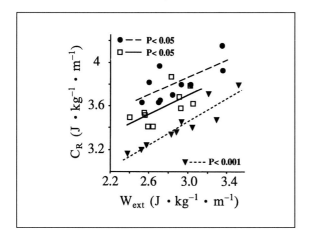

Fig. 2. C_R in relation to the external work of the center of mass (W_{ext}) in unloaded condition at velocities of 3.61 m · s^{-1} (▼) and 5 m · s^{-1} (●) and in loaded conditions at 5 m · s^{-1} (□) obtained in 10 runners. Data from Bourdin [42].

running velocities of 3.61 and 5 m · s^{-1} in normal conditions, and at 5 m · s^{-1} with extra loading of 9.3% body mass. During the different bouts, kinematic arm measurements were performed and averaged on 10 successive steps. Assuming that the belt movements account for the CM movements, it was then possible to compute the potential and the kinetic CM energy changes of the runner from the vertical and the horizontal displacements measured by the KA [34]. C_R was also determined from oxygen uptake measurements.

Significant relationships were obtained between interindividual differences of C_R and EP_{CM} during running (fig. 2) for running velocities of 3.61 and 5 m · s^{-1} in normal conditions and at 5 m · s^{-1} with extra loading of 9.3% body weight [39]. Furthermore, it was demonstrated that the average decrease of 4.6% in C_R observed with vertical loading could be explained by a concomitant 4% decrease in EP_{CM}, and that interindividual changes in C_R and EP_{CM} induced by extra loading were also significantly correlated [39] (fig. 3).

To the best of our knowledge, such relationships were not previously reported in the literature [37, 41]. Applying the KA method to treadmill running allowed the measurements to be performed on a sufficient number of steps which reduced the errors due to step variability. Furthermore, test-retest variability was also reduced by simultaneous measurement of mechanical and metabolic parameters. This could explain that a significant relationship between C_R and EP_{CM} was found with the KA measurement method.

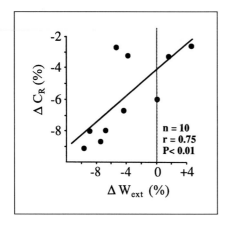

Fig. 3. Variations of C_R between unloaded and loaded conditions (ΔC_R) in relation to the corresponding variations of the external work of the center of mass (ΔW_{ext}). Data from Bourdin [42].

However, this does not mean that the KA measurement method gives the exact value of muscular work. In fact, although the mechanical energy values obtained with the KA lay within the range of values reported in the literature [39, 42], the corresponding mean efficiency value of 76% is higher than 'standard' efficiency values of 40–50% usually found in the literature [9] when only 'external' CM energy is taken into account. This efficiency overestimation is probably not due to the lack of accuracy of the KA by itself [33] but to the fact that the movements measured at the belt level do not exactly account for CM displacements in the horizontal direction. During running, a trunk oscillation occurs in the forward-backward direction [43]. Because the belt is probably located below the rotating point of the trunk [9], this body oscillation is partly measured by the KA. Recent measurements [unpubl. data] have shown that when trunk tilting is measured and taken into account, efficiency values obtained with the KA could decrease to about 40% and thus be compatible with the 'external' CM efficiency found in the literature [9]. Nevertheless, the trunk oscillations are connected with the 'internal' CM mechanical work production. It could then be assumed that the KA method provides a measurement of both external and internal CM mechanical work, which already showed the best relationship with C_R in the literature [37]. It is also worth noting that in treadmill conditions, the intrastep variation of the treadmill belt velocity could also influence the kinetic energy changes of the CM of the runner [44]. These variations were found to be 10% of the belt velocity [38]. However, in a recent study [45, 46], no KA mechanical energy differences were obtained between track and treadmill running.

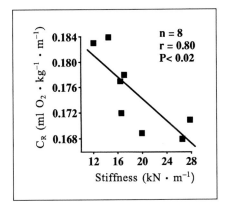

Fig. 4. C_R in relation to the stiffness of the leg determined by the spring-mass model. Data from Dalleau et al. [50].

The Spring Mass Model

Instead of considering the mechanical energy production as the main factor influencing the efficiency of running, an alternate view focuses on the recuperative possibilities of muscles. Cavagna et al. [9] considered the running man as a bouncing ball simply storing and releasing elastic energy during the contact phase. Subsequently, several authors [47–49] have modelised the runner as a simple mechanical model constituted of a mass (the body) oscillating on a spring (the leg). The spring is characterised by its stiffness. Knowing the mass and the stiffness parameters, it is possible to determine the natural frequency of the system at which it oscillates without any production or consumption of mechanical energy.

This model was applied in 8 experienced middle-distance runners [50] running at a velocity corresponding to 90% of their maximal aerobic velocity $(5.1 \pm 0.3 \text{ m} \cdot \text{s}^{-1})$. Their C_R was determined by the open-circuit method. Using the kinematic arm, it was possible to concomitantly measure the displacement and the energy changes of the body during the steps. Assuming that, during the eccentric phase of contact, the measured displacement corresponds to the spring shortening and that the energy changes correspond to the storage of elastic energy, it was possible to calculate the stiffness of the leg and then to determine the natural oscillating frequency of the runner.

The calculated stiffness was in agreement with values previously obtained with methods based on force platform measurements [47, 48]. For the propulsive leg (i.e. the leg producing the highest CM work), there was a significant relationship ($p < 0.02$) between C_R and the stiffness of the leg determined by the spring-mass model (fig. 4). C_R was also significantly related ($p < 0.02$) to the absolute difference between the natural frequency of the spring-mass model

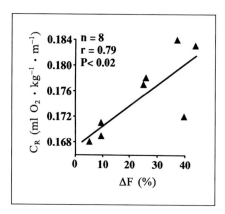

Fig. 5. C_R in relation to the relative difference (ΔF) between the natural oscillation frequency of the spring-mass model (Fn) and the step frequency of the runner (Fr). $\Delta F = |(\mathrm{Fn} - \mathrm{Fr}) \times \mathrm{Fn}^{-1}| \times 100$. Data from Dalleau et al. [50].

and the real step frequency observed during running (fig. 5). However, these relationships were not confirmed for the leg producing less mechanical work. It could be hypothesised that the functional differences previously observed between the legs [38] explain their different influence on C_R. Nevertheless, these results showed that the recuperative properties of the muscles could also influence C_R.

A Treadmill for Force Measurements

The kinetic measurements deal with the same step variability problems as the kinematic measurements [51]. The kinetic parameters of running, i.e. ground reaction forces, are generally obtained in field conditions by means of ground-mounted force platforms. Like video or film analysis, force platforms are expensive and researchers are also limited in the number of successive ground contacts they can measure. On the other hand, in laboratory conditions, treadmills allow metabolic measurements during long running bouts, but they are limited in biomechanical measurements. Kram and Powell [52] proposed to incorporate a force platform under the moving belt of the treadmill. However, this technical solution allowed accurate measurements of the vertical force only.

In order to measure both the vertical and the horizontal ground reaction forces in treadmill conditions, a new type of treadmill was recently designed [53]. The main idea was to mechanically isolate the entire treadmill. For that purpose, all the treadmill components, including the motor, were tightly mounted on a single metal frame. This frame was calculated to be as rigid as possible and was tightly fixed to the ground through crystal force transducers

Belli

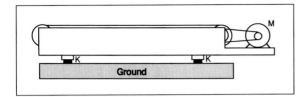

Fig. 6. Schematic side view of the treadmill. K and M indicate the locations of the force transducers and of the motor, respectively. Data from Belli et al. [53].

(fig. 6). In that case, forces due to the treadmill moving parts or to belt friction could be considered as internal forces and only the external forces produced by the subject's feet were measured by the force transducers.

The first prototype was designed for walking measurements. It consisted of two symmetrical parts separated by a 7-mm gap, allowing force measurements of the left and right foot during the double support phase of walking. The static linearity (99.5%) and resonant frequency obtained (> 33 Hz) were acceptable for walking conditions. Furthermore the magnitudes and the directions of forces obtained during normal walking were in agreement with data obtain from ground-mounted force platforms [54].

However, in order to apply this new treadmill concept to force measurements during running, further analysis and trials are in progress in order to obtain stiffer and lighter treadmill frames. Because there is no double support phase in running, better characteristics could probably be obtained by using a single frame mounted on four crystal force transducers. Furthermore, simulation results showed that in this later case a resonant frequency of at least 200 Hz would be a reasonable goal. Therefore, this kind of treadmill could be applied in the future for further calculations of mechanical energy during running, based on both kinematic and kinetic measurements and obtained from a large number of steps.

Conclusion

The exact calculation of the running efficiency is not possible because of the difficulties encountered in defining and measuring the mechanical energy produced by the muscles during running. However, when the mechanical energy of the CM was measured and averaged on a sufficient number of steps by means of a KA, EP_{CM} could be significantly related to C_R. When the same measurement system was applied to define the characteristics of a spring-mass model, the recuperative properties of muscle could also be linked to C_R. Therefore these new methods could provide significant insight into the mechanical variable influencing the efficiency of running. A new treadmill, allowing force measurements on many steps could also help us, in the future, to accurately describe the interaction between mechanical EP and the recuperative properties of the muscles.

References

1   Cavanagh PR, Kram R: The efficiency of human movement – a statement of the problem. Med Sci Sports Exerc 1985;17:304–308.
2   Margaria R: Sulla fisiologica, e specialmente sul consumo ernergetico, della marcia et della corsa a varie velocità ed inclinazione del terreno. Atti Accad Naz Lincei 1938;7:299–368.
3   Åstrand PO, Rodahl K: Energy metabolism and the factors governing the selection of fuel for muscular exercise; in Textbook of Work Physiology, ed 3. New York, McGraw-Hill, 1986, pp 543–556.
4   Di Pramprero PE: The energy cost of human locomotion on land and in water. Int J Sports Med 1986;7:55–72.
5   Lacour J-R: Influence of body dimensions, sex and training on the energy cost of running. Med Sci Sport Sci. Basel, Karger, 1996, vol 41, pp 32–43.
6   Bourdin M, Pastene J, Germain M, Lacour JR: Influence of training, sex, age and body mass on the energy cost of running. Eur J Appl Physiol 1993;66:439–444.
7   Lacour JR, Padilla-Magunacelaya S, Barthelemy JC, Dormois D: The energetics of middle-distance running. Eur J Appl Physiol 1990;61:446–452.
8   Fenn WO: Work against gravity and work due to velocity changes. Am J Physiol 1930;93:433–462.
9   Cavagna GA, Saibene FP, Margaria R: Mechanical work in running. J Appl Physiol 1964;19: 249–256.
10   Winter DA: A new definition of mechanical work done in human movement. J Appl Physiol 1979; 46:79–83.
11   Pierrynowski MR, Winter DA, Norman RW: Transfers of mechanical energy within the total body and mechanical efficiency during treadmill running. Ergonomics 1980;23:147–156.
12   Aleshinsky SY: An energy 'sources' and 'fractions' approach to the mechanical energy expenditure problem I. Basic concepts, description of the model, analysis of a one link system movement. J Biomech 1986;19:288–293.
13   Aleshinsky SY: An energy 'sources' and 'fractions' approach to the mechanical energy expenditure problem. II. Movement of the multi-link chain model. J Biomech 1986;19:295–300.
14   Aleshinsky SY: An energy 'sources' and 'fractions' approach to the mechanical energy expenditure problem. IV. Criticism of the concept of 'energy transfers' within and between links. J Biomech 1986;19:307–309.
15   Elftman H: Forces and energy changes in the leg during walking. Am J Physiol 1939;125:337–366.
16   Wells RP: Mechanical energy cost of human movements: An approach to evaluating the transfer possibilities of two-joints muscles. J Biomech 1988;21:955–964.
17   Hatze H: The complete optimisation of human motion. Math Biol Sci 1976;28:99–135.
18   Pandy MG, Anderson FC, Hull DG: A parameter optimization approach for the optimal control of large-scale musculoskeletal systems. J Biomech Engin 1992;114:450–460.
19   Belli A, Bosco C: Influence of stretch-shortening cycle on mechanical behaviour of triceps surae during hopping. Acta Physiol Scand 1992;144:401–408.
20   Komi PV, Belli A, Huttunen V, Partio E: Optic fiber as a transducer for direct in-vivo measurements of human tendomuscular forces; Proceedings of the XVth Congress of the International Society of Biomechanics, Jyväskylä, July 2–6, 1995, pp 494–495.

21   Davies CTM: The effect of wind assistance and resistance on the forward motion of a runner. J Appl Physiol 1980;48:702–709.

22   Cavagna GA, Dusman B, Margaria R: Positive work done by a previously stretched muscle. J Appl Physiol 1968:24:21–32.

23   Goubel F: Muscle mechanics. Fundamental concepts in stretch-shortening cycle. Med Sport Sci 1987;26:24–35.

24   Komi PV: Stretch-shortening cycle; in Komi PV (ed): Strength and Power in Sport. IOC Medical Commission Publication. Oxford, Blackwell, 1992, pp 169–179.

25   Komi PV, Kyröläinen H: Mechanical efficiency of stretch-shortening cycle exercise. Med Sci Sport Sci. Basel, Karger, 1996, vol 41, pp 44–56.

26   Asmussen E, Bonde Petersen F: Apparent efficiency and storage of elastic energy in human muscles during exercise. Acta Physiol Scand 1974;92:537–545.

27   Lensel-Corbeil G, Goubel F: Series elasticity in frog sartorius muscle subjected to stretch-shortening cycles. J Biomech 1990;23:121–126.

28   Aura O, Komi PV: Effects of pre-stretch intensity on mechanical efficiency of positive work and on elastic behaviour of skeletal muscle in stretch-shortening cycle exercise. Int J Sports Med 1986;7:137–143.

29   Bosco C, Tihanyi J, Komi PV, Fekete G, Apor P: Store and recoil of elastic energy in slow and fast types of human skeletal muscle. Acta Physiol Scand 1982;116:343–349.

30   Aura O, Komi PV: Effect of muscle fibre distribution on the mechanical efficiency of human locomotion. Int J Sports Med 1987;S8:30–37.

31   Williams KR: The relationship between mechanical and physiological energy estimates. Med Sci Sports Exerc 1985;17:317–325.

32   Kaneko M: Mechanics and energetics in running with special reference to efficiency. J Biomech 1990;23S1:57–63.

33   Belli A, Rey S, Bonnefoy R, Lacour JR: A simple device for kinematic measurements of human movement. Ergonomics 1992;35:177–186.

34   Belli A, Avela J, Komi PV: Mechanical energy assessment with different methods during running. Int J Sports Med 1993;14:252–256.

35   Williams KR, Cavanagh PR: Relationship between distance running mechanics, running economy and performance. J Appl Physiol 1987;63:1236–1245.

36   Morgan DW, Martin PE, Krähenbühl GS: Factors affecting running economy. Sports Med 1989; 7:310–330.

37   Martin PE, Heise GD, Morgan DW: Interrelationships between mechanical power, energy transfers, and walking and running economy. Med Sci Sports Exerc 1993;25:508–515.

38   Belli A, Lacour JR, Komi PV, Candau R, Denis C: Mechanical step variability during treadmill running. Eur J Appl Physiol 1995;70:510–517.

39   Bourdin M, Belli A, Arsac LM, Bosco C, Lacour JR: Effect of vertical loading on energy cost and kinematics of running in trained male subjects. J Appl Physiol, in press.

40   Bourdin M, Belli A, Arsac LM, Bosco C, Lacour JR: Effect of velocity on mechanics and energy cost of running; in Proceedings of the XVth Congress of the International Society of Biomechanics, Jyväskylä, July 2–6, 1995, pp 124–125.

41   Shorten MR, Wooton SA, Williams C: Mechanical energy changes and the oxygen cost of running. Engin Med 1981;10:213–217.

42   Bourdin M: Facteurs mécaniques et neuro-musculaires de variation du coût énergétique de la course à pied; thèse, Université Lyon I, Lyon, 1995.

43   Thorstensson A, Nilsson J, Carlson H, Zomlefer MR: Trunk movements in human locomotion. Acta Physiol Scand 1984;121:9–22.

44   Van Ingen Schenau GJ: Some fundamental aspects of the biomechanics of overgound versus treadmill locomotion. Med Sci Sports Exerc 1980;12:257–261.

45   Kyröläinen H, Komi PV, Belli A: Mechanical efficiency in athletes during running. Scand J Med Sci Sports 1995;5:200–208.

46   Belli A, Kyröläinen H, Komi PV: Mechanical efficiency comparison between treadmill and track running (abstract) 42nd Meeting of the American College of Sports Medicine. Med Sci Sports Exerc 1995;27(suppl):S162.

Mechanical Factors of Running Efficiency

47   Luhtanen P, Komi PV: Force-, power-, and elasticity-velocity relationships in walking, running and jumping. Eur J Appl Physiol 1980;44:279–289.

48   Blickhan R: The spring-mass model for running and hopping. J Biomech 1989;22:1217–1227.

49   McMahon TA, Cheng GC: The mechanics of running: How does stiffness couple with speed? J Biomechanics 1990;23:65–78.

50   Dalleau G, Belli A, Bourdin M, Lacour JR: Energy cost and spring mass model in human running; in Proceedings of the XVth Congress of the International Society of Biomechanics, Jyväskylä, July 2–6, 1995, pp 196–197.

51   Bates BT, Osternig LR, Mason BR, James SL: Functional variability of lower extremity during the support phase of running. Med Sci Sports Exerc 1979;11:328–331.

52   Kram R, Powell AJ: A treadmill mounted force platform. J Appl Physiol 1989;67:1692–1698.

53   Belli A, Bui P, Berger A, Lacour JR: A treadmill for measurement of ground reaction forces during walking; in Proceedings of the XVth Congress of the International Society of Biomechanics, Jyväskylä, July 2–6, 1995, pp 100–101.

54   Nilsson J, Thorstensson A: Ground reaction forces at different speeds of human walking and running. Acta Physiol Scand 1989;136:217–227.

Alain Belli, Laboratoire de Physiologie de l'Exercice, Faculté de Médecine Lyon-Sud,
Chemin du Petit-Revoyet, BP 12, F–69921 Oullins Cédex (France)

Marconnet P, Saltin B, Komi P, Poortmans J (eds): Human Muscular Function
during Dynamic Exercise. Med Sport Sci. Basel, Karger, 1996, vol 41, pp 71–81

....

Is Electrical Stimulation Applicable to Improve Strength and Power in Normal Humans?

Gary A. Dudley

Department of Exercise Science, University of Georgia, Athens, GA., USA

Introduction

There is little doubt that improved training techniques have had much to do with enhanced athletic performance over the past few decades. Coaches, trainers, athletes and scientists conduct a never-ending search for the conditioning program that will result in the ultimate performance. One such approach that has begun to gain renewed interest is surface electrical stimulation (SES). You are probably familiar with SES in regard to its application in rehabilitation medicine. When activation of skeletal muscle by voluntary means is compromised, SES has been used to either control deterioration of neuromuscular function after injury or enhance recovery [e.g.1–5]. You may be somewhat unaware of the fact that SES is also receiving increased use in basic research concerning human skeletal muscle metabolism and mechanical function. Hultman's group [e.g. 6, 7] has conducted numerous studies of human muscle metabolism using the biopsy technique combined with SES. Several others have also used SES in recent years to study mechanical characteristics of human skeletal muscle in vivo [e.g. 8–14]. Most recently, SES has been combined with ^{31}P magnetic resonance spectrocopy for in vivo studies of human muscle metabolism [e.g. 15]. One general observation that arises from these studies is that SES can be used to evoke forceful muscle actions that dictate a marked increase in energy turnover of the stimulated muscle. With these responses to SES now clearly documented, it is not surprising that interest in the use of artificial activation as a conditioning tool by athletes has risen in recent years. This brief paper will describe application of SES, differences in muscle actions evoked by SES versus voluntary effort, probable exploration of these differences for advantageous use of SES in conditioning of athletes, data supporting SES use in athletes and future research directions.

Application of SES

A large variety of commercially available electrical stimulation units exist today, mainly put forth by medical equipment suppliers. These in large part possess a variety of 'set' stimulation protocols, from which the one of choice can be selected. It should be appreciated that these different protocols in general are designed with rehabilitation in mind. They generally consist of a 'long' ramp time, that is, a gradual increase in amplitude, stimulation at a frequency that evokes tetani or near tetani, a duration of the train of pulses that is generally several seconds long, a duty cycle of 1 to 1 or much greater and a pulse duration that is usually less than 250 µs.

A variety of different electrodes are available, but irrespective of their make-up, the negative one is usually placed over the motor point, the location where greatest force arises for a given stimulation paradigm, and the positive one is placed far removed from its counterpart on the muscle group of interest [16]. Force development via SES increases with electrode size [17], and it is best to have the electrodes in place several minutes before SES in an effort to allow insensible perspiration to accumulate at the electrode-skin interface to minimize hot spots [18].

OK, we are now set up to apply SES to a willing subject, so let us turn on the switch. But first, how should we set up our protocol? How do pulse duration, frequency and stimulation amplitude effect force development? It seems our interest, especially with regard to strength and power athletes, should be to maximize force output while minimizing fatigue. Force arising from SES increases as pulse frequency increases up to about 500µs and thereafter plateaus [19]. Hultman et al. [19] have, thus, put forth that optimal pulse duration should be between 500 and 1,000 µs. Force arising from SES also increases in a sigmoidal relation with pulse frequency and stimulation amplitude [20]. Pulse frequencies of about 50 per second (Hz) or greater evoke tetanus, and thereby optimal force output of stimulated muscle [20]. As it turns out, amplitude is often limited by subject tolerance. In light of these observations, it is surprising that commercial SES devices seldom deliver pulses with a duration greater that 250 µs. This would be expected to limit force for a given SES protocol because of the steep, positive relation between pulse duration and force. Little is known about the effect of different wave forms on SES, but it seems that those bipolar in nature are most tolerable. So, what does our stimulation protocol look like? Suppose we want to stimulate the quadriceps femoris muscle group. One electrode would be placed over the proximal aspect to the vastus lateralis muscle, the other over the distal aspect of the vastus medialis muscle. About 15 min after electrode placement, SES consisting of 500 µs, sigmoidal pulses delivered at 50 Hz for 500 to 1,000 ms would be used to evoke a single, tetanic muscle action. Oh, two other notes. First, resistance to movement should be used during SES to maximize force development and limit shortening. Intensity of conditioning, as judged by the training load or in the case of SES force developed, is the most important factor for inducing adaptive responses to 'resistance' training [21]. Application of resistance will also limit muscle shortening, and thereby maintain organization of contractile machinery [22]. Most often, isometric actions are evoked, but more recently SES has been applied during lengthening and/or shortening actions [9–11,13,14]. SES is generally applied in lieu of voluntary effort, but the two have been combined [23]. And second, a train duration of 500–1,000 ms was chosen because time to peak tension for an SES evoked tetanic, isometric action is 250 ms for this muscle group [9, 11]. Thus, we are providing ample time for optimization of external force development without causing undue fatigue during each muscle action.

Characteristics of SES versus Voluntary Effort

There seem to be three major differences between muscle actions evoked by SES versus voluntary effort with regard to muscle fiber recruitment: namely the frequency, synchrony and order of motor units recruitment. Motor unit recruitment during voluntary effort is generally held to follow the 'size principle' although there are a few noted exceptions [24–26]. Thus, slow, fatigue-resistant motor units are recruited first during voluntary effort, and fast, less fatigue-resistant units are brought into play as force is increased. Variations in motor unit firing frequency and/or in the number of motor units employed are used to achieve increments in force depending on the size and fiber type composition of the muscle [27, 28]. A second strategy is also used to optimize force development while minimizing fatigue during voluntary effort. Motor units are recruited in a more or less asynchronous manner [29, 30]. In this way, less energy is used in 'tightening up' the elastic elements in muscle, thereby requiring less energy turnover for a given external force development.

SES, in contrast, activates a given portion of muscle in a synchronous manner. This could, in part, explain the greater fatigue traditionally noticed with SES versus voluntary effort [8, 12]. SES is also generally applied at frequencies designed to evoke tetani of fast motor units, for example 50 Hz. This is essentially 'over-kill' for slow motor units where fusion frequency is below 25 Hz [27, 28]. The higher frequency is used to ensure tetani, and thereby, optimal force development of fast motor units. However, fast motor units are seldom activated at 50 Hz or more during voluntary effort, save for brief periods [27, 28]. In fact, it is generally held that sedentary individuals have extreme difficulty in achieving such activation of fast motor units [27, 28]. This high frequency of activation with SES may result in fusion for even the 'fastest' fast units. Owing to such force, however, is an extreme energy demand which may also account for the greater fatigue with SES versus voluntary effort.

Force increments with SES are usually achieved by increasing the amplitude, not frequency of stimulation. The finding that the area of muscle showing contractile-induced contrast shift in proton-weighted magnetic resonance images was positively related to isometric force during SES of the quadriceps femoris muscle group suggests that increases in SES amplitude result in ever increasing amounts of muscle being stimulated [8]. Interestingly, both superficial and deep muscle showed such contrast shift even at low levels of SES. Moreover, the pattern of muscle activation by SES varied markedly among subjects. This leads to a major topic of controversy concerning the application of SES, namely whether this mode of artificial activation leads to an altered pattern of motor unit recruitment, or, as is sometimes suggested, a reverse order of recruitment of motor units. It is often put forth that SES preferentially activates fast motor units because they are served by large motor neurons, that because of their size, are easily depolarized [31–33]. SES is also thought to stimulate cutaneous afferents that inhibit voluntary activation of slow motor units and facilitate excitation of motoneurones of fast motor units [34]. However, SES activates distal motor neurons [19]. How reflex inhibition of slow motorneurones could override this distal activation is not clear. DeLuca's group [35] has found that mean and median frequency and conduction velocity increase with force in a similar mannner for both SES and voluntary effort. Because these variables increase in proportion to fast fiber recruitment, the results were interpreted to suggest that SES does not reverse the normal order of motor unit activation. The authors suggested that this may have occurred because large motorneurones may not necessarily have large branches and/or that orientation of such branches may not have favored their stimulation. In contrast to these findings, Sinacore et al. [36] reported in a case study that SES caused a reversal of the normal recruitment pattern because fast fibers showed preferential glycogen depletion. In a more elaborate study, Saltin et al. [37] reported that SES of the quadriceps femoris muscle group during dynamic knee extension exercise resulted in glycogen depletion of both slow and fast fibers. When voluntary exercise was performed at the same work rate (30 w) and duration (60 min), glycogen depletion occurred only in slow fibers. Thus, it seems that SES activates both slow and fast fibers, probably not reversing the normal order of recruitment. However, the non-discriminate activation of both fast and slow fibers by SES to achieve the same work rate is clearly not advatageous from a metabolic perspective. The relatively greater reliance on fast fibers and the synchronous activation of both fiber types would be expected to exaggerate metabolic demand as compared to performing the same exercise voluntarily with slow fibers recruited in an asynchronous manner. This recruitment strategy for voluntary exercise minimizes the energy demand of force maintenance while taking advantage of the great ability of slow fibers to supply energy for contraction.

The end result of the activation of skeletal muscle is force development. What might one expect to be different between SES and voluntary efforts regarding the mechanical characteristics of force development? As noted previously, the ability to maintain force for a given time-tension integral is much less with SES. For example, untrained subjects can maintain force during voluntary isometric knee extensions at forces up to 75% of maximal voluntary when efforts are performed with a 1 s/1 s duty cycle. When the same force is generated by SES and repeat muscle actions are evoked with the same work/rest cycle, fatigue of 10–15% occurs after 10 or so actions [8]. The rise time to peak tension during isometric efforts is not overly different between tetanic SES and maximal voluntary efforts [9]. About 250 ms are needed to realize a plateau in force. It is not known whether relaxation is markedly different between these modes of muscle activation, but suffice it to suggest that the greater fatigue with SES probably arises from its synchronous activation of muscle fibers and greater reliance on fast fibers.

Several laboratories have used voluntary effort or SES to examine the speed-torque relation of human skeletal muscle in vivo. Edgerton's group [38–41] has clearly shown that force is less for slow, shortening voluntary efforts than can be produced by skeletal muscle stimulated in vitro, and suggested that some neural inhibitory mechanisms limit force during such actions. Others have reported similar results, some even extending these observations to lengthening actions [9,11,42,43]. Taken together, they imply that force varies much less as a function of speed of action for voluntary effort than can be realized when skeletal muscle is activated in vitro. Why this apparent damping of force is evident for volunteer effort is not clear, but it has been suggested that this may serve to minimize trauma, especially during lengthening actions. A few groups have recently used SES to study human muscle mechanics in vivo with much the same result [9,11,13,14]. They found that (1) force varied as a function of speed to a much greater extent for SES that for voluntary efforts, (2) in vivo mechanical characteristics of human skeletal muscle are quite comparable to those of muscle studied in vitro and (3) SES-evoked forces per unit of muscle can be much greater than those arising from voluntary effort, especially for lengthening actions.

Probable Uses of SES in Conditioning

Based on the aforementioned presentation, several probable uses of SES in conditioning can be envisioned. Most notable, activation of fast muscle at fusion frequency (about 50Hz) seems attractive, especially because untrained individuals have extreme difficulty in activating these high-threshold units. This would be expected to impose mechanical loading on these units seldom achieved by voluntary effort, at least until fatigue. SES could also be used to impose substantial loading on skeletal muscle, especially during lengthening actions, by by-passing some neural factors that appear to limit force during voluntary effort. The marked metabolic demand that arises from SES could also be used for endurance training.

Data Supporting SES in Conditioning

The use of SES in conditioning in healthy individuals, particularly athletes, began receiving attention in the early 1970s based on the work of Kots and Chwilon [44]. They originally suggested that SES after 4–5 weeks could increase strength 30–40%. Their explanation for this impressive improvement seems to arise from the observation that SES forces were 10–30% greater than maximal voluntary, thereby providing greater loading to evoke adaptions to training. Unfortunately, neither force data during SES nor measures of muscle size were reported. Later work by Kots and colleagues failed to duplicate these findings [45]. They showed little or no change in muscle size or strength after 7 sessions of SES applied over 8 days. These data do not necessarily fail to establish the efficacy of SES conditioning, however. Increasing muscle size and strength in athletes with almost any modality in such a short time would seem quite difficult.

Delitto et al. [46] have provided data to suggest that SES may have particular benefit in conditioning strength/power athletes. They applied SES to the quadriceps femoris muscle group of an elite lifter at an amplitude that evoked force equal to 112% of maximal voluntary isometric. SES was applied 3 days each week during weeks 5–8 and weeks 13 and 14 of the lifter's regular training. Ten 11-second contractions were applied each day. Over the course of these 14 weeks of training, the lifter showed a 20-kg increase in the 1 repetition maximum for the squat, and also showed increases for the clean and jerk, and snatch. The 20-kg increase in the squat is striking considering the observation that elite lifters do not generally show such increases over 2 years of regular training [47]. What are the possible explanations for such an increase? Average fiber size in biopsies of the vastus lateralis appeared to decrease over training, thus hypertrophy does not seem to be the answer. Hyperplasia could have occurred to increase muscle size, but whether this arises as a result of over-load training is controversial [48], and no measures of whole muscle cross-sectional area were made in this case study, so the authors could not estimate fiber number. Finally, no estimates of muscle activation or lifting technique were made, thus it is not known whether enhanced motor control could explain the improvement.

We have recently examined the effect of 9 weeks of SES on thigh muscle growth when lengthening and shortening actions were performed in lieu of more traditional isometric actions [49]. SES was applied to the left quadriceps femoris muscle group of 8 trainees while 8 additional subjects trained the same muscle group using voluntary effort. The right quadriceps femoris muscle group served as an internal 'control' in each group. Subjects trained 2 days each week, with 3–5 sets of 10 coupled lengthening and shortening actions being performed. SES amplitude was set to induce an isometric torque equal to 70–80% of maximal voluntary. Magnetic resonance images taken before and after SES conditioning showed a 10% increase in average cross-sectional area of the left quadriceps femoris muscle group in SES trainees, while subjects using voluntary efforts showed a 4% increase. Neither group showed a change in average cross-sectional area of the right quadriceps femoris muscle group. When statistics were applied to these data, there was significant interaction, suggesting that SES evoked greater hypertrophy than voluntary conditioning.

It would seem that these aforementioned results support the use of SES in conditioning, even of athletes. However, it should be appreciated that our recent work was conducted using untrained subjects. Our interest arose from the general observation that enhanced performance during the early course of resistance training has been ascribed to neural adaptations, with hypertrophy becoming the more dominant factor as training proceeds [50]. We were interested in seeing whether the neural inhibitory factors that compromise force during 'maximal' voluntary efforts might limit hypertrophy during the early course of resistance training. Thus, it seemed reasonable to bypass voluntary activation by using SES. We also made the decision to use lengthening actions in an effort to maximize loading during SES as opposed to voluntary effort where neural factors markedly compromise force. Our results are quite encouraging for the application of SES to conditioning of strength/power athletes.

These individuals, however, have been conditioning for years, and thus have enjoyed marked adaptations to training [47, 50]. They characteristically show preferential fast-fiber hypertrophy and specific tension, even when corrected for muscle size, that is much greater than that of untrained individuals [21, 51]. Thus, they have enjoyed substantial neural adaptions to conditioning and can clearly activate fast fibers to the extent that impressive growth is realized. It is not clear that the potential benefits of SES, including extensive activation of fast fiber, would impose greater loading that the regular conditioning performed by strength/power athletes.

Recent research has shown that 3 h per day of 5–10 Hz SES applied for 6 weeks increases resistance to fatigue and skeletal muscle aerobic-oxidative enzyme content of lower limb muscle groups in untrained individuals [52, 53]. The magnitude of the increase in enzyme content was less than that reported previously for chronic stimulation of skeletal muscle of lower mammals for the same duration and failed to result in enzyme activities comparable to those of elite athletes. The authors suggested, therefore, that surface SES in humans may not provide a stimulus comparable to chronic nerve stimulation in lower mammals, or that the potential for mitochrondrial biogenesis is less in human skeletal muscle than that of lower mammals. However, the fact that SES was applied during the course of daily activities would suggest that force development was not optimal, and this could have limited energy demand and thereby metabolic adaptation.

Future Directions

It is clear that some neural inhibitory mechanisms limit force during voluntary eccentric actions. The extent to which this inhibition has been overcome by years of heavy-resistance training, typically performed by strength/power athletes, is not known. Their high specific tension and impressive fast-fiber size would suggest that neural inhibitory mechanisms limit force much less in elite lifters as compared to untrained individuals. Nevertheless, it would be interesting to determine whether SES, applied during voluntary muscle actions, could evoke even greater hypertrophy in these athletes. It might be that SES could more fully activate slow fibers during eccentric actions, where neural factors are suggested to limit their use [25,26]. It would also be of interest to determine the effect of long-term, more chronic SES on the aerobic-oxidative enzyme capacity of human skeletal muscle. Application of SES in this manner in lower mammals has been shown to evoke impressive increases in the ability of skeletal muscle to supply energy by aerobic means [54]. This chronic application of SES would need to be done with caution, however, because it may also evoke muscle fiber degeneration and atrophy, results not especially appealing to athletes [55].

Minimizing the discomfort of SES will also need to be addressed, although some individuals are quite tolerant. It is possible to evoke forces near maximal voluntary when applying SES to large muscle groups, such as the knee extensors, although this has been questioned [1, 8, 9, 11, 14, 49, 56]. Force arising from stimulating smaller muscle groups, for example, the forearm flexors, that may be important in athletic performance, in contrast, have been reported to be about one third of maximal [23].

Acknowledgments

My colleagues, Paul Buchanan and Marc Duvoisin, are gratefully acknowledged for introducing me to the topic of electromyostimulation and its hardware, and many insightful discussions on these issues. My work cited herein was supported in part by grants from the National Aeronautic and Space Administration administered under contracts NAS 10 10285 and NAS10 11624.

References

1   Delitto A, Robinson AF: Electrical stimulation of muscle: Techniques and applications; in Snyder-Mackler L, Robinson AJ (eds): Clinical Electrophysiology: Electrotherapy and Electrophysiologic Testing. Baltimore, Williams & Wilkins, 1989, pp95–138.
2   Eriksson E, Haggmark T: Comparison of isometric muscle training and electrical stimulation supplementing isometric muscle training in the recovery after major knee ligament surgery. Am J Sports Med 1979;169–171.
3   Gordon T, Mao J: Muscle atrophy and procedures for training after spinal cord injury. Phys Ther 1994;74:56–66.
4   Johnson DH, Thurston P, Ashcroft PJ: The Russian technique of faradism in the treatment of chondromalacia patellae. Physiother Canada 1977;29:266–268.
5   Wigerstad-Lossing I, Grimby G, Jonsson T, Morelli B, Peterson L, Renstrom P: Effects of electrical muscle stimulation combined with voluntary contractions after knee ligament surgery. Med Sci Sport Exerc 1988;20:93–98.
6   Hultman E, Sjoholm H: Energy metabolism and contraction force of human skeletal muscle in situ during electrical stimulation. J Appl Physiol 1983;345:525–532.
7   Constantin-Teodosiu D, Cederblad G, Hultman E: PDC activity and acetyl group accumulation in skeletal muscle during isometric contraction. J Appl Physiol 1993;74:1712–1718.
8   Adams GR, Harris RT, Woodard D, Dudley GA: Mapping of electrical muscle stimulation using MRI. J Appl Physiol 1993;74:532–537.
9   Dudley, GA, Harris RT, Duvoisin MR, Hather BM, Buchanan P: Effect of voluntary vs artificial activation on the relationship of muscle torque to speed. J Appl Physiol 1990;69:2215–2221.
10 Gravel D, Belanger AY, Richards CL: Study of human muscle contraction using electrically evoked twitch responses during passive shortening and lengthening movements. Eur J Appl Physiol 1987; 56:623–627.
11 Harris RT, Dudley GA: Factors limiting force during slow, shortening actions of the quadriceps femoris muscle group in vivo. Acta Physiol Scand 1994;152:63–71.

12 Lieber RK, Kelly MJ: Torque history of electrically stimulated human quadriceps: Implications for stimulation therapy. J Orthop Res 1993; 11:131–141.

13 Thomas DO, White MJ, Sagar G, Davies CTM: Electrically evoked isokinetic plantar flexor torque in males. J Appl Physiol 1987;63:1499–1503.

14 Westing SH, Seger Jy, Thorstensson A: Effects of electrical stimulation on eccentric and concentric torque-velocity relationships during knee extension in man. Act Physiol Scand 1990;140: 17–22.

15 Blei ML, Conley KE, Odderson IR, Esselman PC, Kushmerick MJ: Individual variation in contractile cost and recovery in human skeletal muscle. Proc Nate Acad Sci USA 1993;90:7396–7400.

16 Ferguson JP, Blackley MW, Knight RD, Sutlive TG, Underwood FB, Greathouse DG: Effects of varying electrode site placements on the torque output of an electrically stimulated involuntary quadriceps femoris muscle contraction. J Orthop Sports Phys Ther 1989;11:24–29.

17 Alon G: High voltage stimulation: Effects of electrode size on basic excitatory responses. Phys Ther 1985;65:890–895.

18 Mason JL,Mackay NAM: Pain sensations associated with electrocutaneous stimulation. IEEE Trans Biomed Eng 1976;23:405–409.

19 Hultman E, Sjoholm H, Jaderholm-Ek I, Krynicki J: Evaluation of methods for electrical stimulation of human skeletal muscle in situ. Pflügers Arch 1983;398:139–141.

20 Davies CTM, Dooley P, McDonagh MJN, White MJ: Adaptation of mechanical properties of muscle to high force training in man. J Physiol (Lond) 1985;365:277–284.

21 Hakkinen K, Keskinen KL: Muscle cross-sectional area and voluntary force production characteristics in elite strength- and endurance-trained athletes and sprinters. Eur J Appl Physiol Occup Physiol 1989;:215–220.

22 Jakubiec-Puka A, Carraro U: Remodelling of the contractile apparatus of striated muscle stimulated electrically in a shortened position. J Anat 1991;178:83–100.

23 Hortobagyi T, Lambert NJ, Tracy C, Shinebarger M: Voluntary and eletromyostimulation forces in trained and untrained men. Med Sci Sports Exerc 1992;24:702–707.

24 Henneman E, Somjen G, Carpenter DO: Functional significance of cell size in spinal motor neurones. J Neurophysiol 1965;28:560–580.

25 Nardone A, Romano C, Schiepatti M: Selective recruitment of high threshold human motor units during voluntary isotonic lengthening of active muscles. J Physiol (Lond) 1989;409:451–471.

26 Nardone A, Schiepatti M: Shift of activity from slow to fast muscle during voluntary lengthening contractions of the triceps surae muscles in humans. J Physiol (Lond) 1988;395:363–381.

27 Basmajian JV, DeLuca CJ: Muscles Alive: Their Functions Revealed by Electromyography. Baltimore, Williams & Wilkins, 1985.

28 Bellemare F, Woods JJ, Johansson R, Bigland-Ritchie B: Motor unit discharge rates in maximal voluntary contractions of three human muscles. J Neurophysiol 1983;50:1380–1392.

29 Clamann HP, Schelhorn TB: Nonlinear force addition of newly recruited motor units in the cat hindlimb. Muscle Nerve 1988;11:1079–1089.

30 Lind AR, Petrofsky JS: Isometric tension from rotary stimulation of fast and slow cat muscles. Muscle Nerve 1987;1:213–218.

31 Delitto A, Snyder-Mackler L: Two theories of muscle strength augmentation using percutaneous electrical stimulation. Phys Ther 1990;70:158–164.

32 Enoka RM: Muscle strength and its development, new perspectives. Sports Med 1988;6:146–168.

33 Solomonow M, Baratta R, Shoji H, D'Ambrosia R: The myoelectric signal of electrically stimulated muscle during recruitment: An inherent feedback parameter for a closed loop control scheme. IEEE Trans Biomed Eng 1986;33:735–745.

34 Garnett R, Stephens JA: Changes in the recruitment threshold of motor units produced by cutaneous stimulation in man. J Physiol (Lond) 1981;311:463–473.

35 Knaflitz M, Merletti R, DeLuca CJ: Inference of motor unit recruitment order in voluntary and electrically elicited contractions. J Appl Physiol 1990;68:1657–1667.

36 Sinacore DR, Delitto A, King DS, Rose SJ: Type II fiber activation with electrical stimulation: A preliminary report. Phys Ther 1990;70:416–422.

Dudley

37   Saltin B, Strange S, Bansbo J, Kim CK, Duvoisin M, Hargens A, Gollnick PD: Central and peripheral cardiovascular adaptations to electrically induced and voluntary exercise. Proc 4th Eur Symp Life Sci Res Space 1990; ESA SP-307:591–595.

38   Caiozzo VR, Perrine JJ, Edgerton VR: Training induced alterations of the in vivo force-velocity relationship of human muscle. J Appl Physiol 1981;51:750–754.

39   Gregor RJ, Edgerton VR, Perrine JJ, Campion DS, DeBus C: Torque-velocity relationships and muscle fiber compositon in elite female athletes. J Appl Physiol 1979;47:388–392.

40   Perrine JJ, Edgerton VR: Muscle force-velocity and power-velocity relationships under isokinetic loading. Med Sci Sports 1978;10:159–166.

41   Wickiewicz TL, Roy RR, Powell PL, Perrine JJ, Edgerton VR: Muscle architecture and force-velocity relationships in humans. J Appl Physiol 1984;57:435–443.

42   Colliander EB, Tesch PA: Bilateral eccentric and concentric torque of quadriceps and hamstring muscles in females and males. Eur J Appl Physiol 1989;59:227–232.

43   Westing SH, Cresswell AG, Thorstensson A: Muscle activation during maximal voluntary eccentric and concentric knee extension. Eur J Appl Physiol 1991;62:104–108.

44   Kots Y, Chwilon W: Muscle training with the electrical stimulation method. Teor Prakt Fizicheskoi Kultury USSR 1971;3/4.

45   St Pierre D, Taylor AW Lavoie M, Sellers W, Kots YM: Effects of 2500 Hz sinusoidal current on fibre area and strength of the quadriceps femoris. J Sports Med 1986;26:60–66.

46   Delitto A, Brown M, Strube MJ, Rose SJ, Lehman RC: Electrical stimulation of quadriceps femoris in an elite weight lifter: A single subject experiment. Int J Sports Med 1989;10:187–191.

47   Hakkinen K, Pakarinen A, Alen M, Kauhanen H, Komi PV: Neuromuscular and hormonal adaptations in athletes to strength training in two years. J Appl Physiol 1988;65:2406–2412.

48   MacDougall JD: Hypertrophy or hyperplasia, in Komi P (ed): Strength and Power in Sport. London, Blackwell, 1992, pp 230–238.

49   Ruther CL, Golden CL, Harris RT, Dudley GA: Hypertrophy, resistance training and the nature of skeletal muscle activation. J Strength Cond Res 1995;9:155–159.

50   Komi PV: Training of muscle strength and power: Interaction of neuromotoric, hypertrophic, and mechanical factors. Int J Sports Med 1986;7:10–15.

51   Ryushi T, Hakkinen K, Kauhanen H, Komi PV: Muscle fiber characteristics, muscle cross-sectional area and force production in strength athletes, physically active males and females. Scand J Sports Sci 1988;10:7–15.

52   Gauthier JM, Theriault R, Theriault G, Gelinas Y, Simoneau JA: Electrical stimulation-induced changes in skeletal muscle enzymes of men and women. Med Sci Sports Exerc 1992;24:1252–1256.

53   Scott OM, Vrbova G, Hyde SA, Dubowitz V: Effects of chronic low frequency electrical stimulation on normal human tibialis anterior muscle. J Neurol Neurosurg Psychiatry 1985;48:774-781.

54   Pette D, Vrbova G: Invited review: Neural control of phenotypic expression in mammalian muscle fibers. Muscle Nerve 1985;8:676–689.

55   Maier A, Gambke B, Pette D: Degeneration-regeneration as a mechanism contributing to the fast to slow conversion of chronically stimulated fast-twich rabbit muscle. Cell Tissue Res 1986;244:635–643.

56   Lieber RL, Kelly J: Factors influencing quadriceps torque using transcutaneous electrical stimulation. Phys Ther 1991;71:715–721.

Gary T. Dudley, PhD, Department of Exercise Science, The University of Georgia, Athens, GA 30602 (USA)

Marconnet P, Saltin B, Komi P, Poortmans J (eds): Human Muscular Function
during Dynamic Exercise. Med Sport Sci. Basel, Karger, 1996, vol 41, pp 82–94

....

The Muscle Contractile System and Its Adaptation to Training

Stephen D.R. Harridge

Copenhagen Muscle Research Centre, Rigshospitalet, Denmark

Muscle Contraction and Myosin Isoform Expression

Muscle contracts through the interaction of interdigitating protein fila-
ments, a mechanism which is powered by the hydrolysis of ATP at the level
of individual cross-bridge sites. Of all the factors which are involved in this
process this paper will focus on the properties of myosin, the contractile
protein of the thick filament which has been shown to be a key factor
regulating the shortening properties of skeletal muscle fibres [1–4]. The functional properties of skeletal muscle, in terms of its force-velocity relationship
are summarised in figure 1. As the velocity of contraction increases, the force-
generating capacity falls until it reaches zero and the velocity of shortening is
at its maximum (V_0). The product of force and velocity is power, with peak
power production occurring at $\sim 30\%$ of V_0 [5]. Thus to increase its power-
generating potential, a muscle has to either increase its force-generating
capacity, or to increase the velocity at which it can shorten. Muscle force
production can be increased through increasing its size (hypertrophy). This
can be brought about by increased chronic mechanical loading, i.e. resistance
or weight training, although the precise mechanisms governing this are still
unclear. Theoretically, to alter the speed at which a muscle can shorten, it
has to either alter its length (change the number of sarcomeres in series) or
alter the contractile proteins it expresses. The latter of these mechanisms will
be focused on here.

A myosin molecule (shown schematically in fig. 2) is composed of two
heavy-chain (MHC) components which comprise a head and tail region each
with a molecular weight of ~ 200 kD. Associated with each MHC are two
myosin light chains (MLC; ~ 25 kD each). The subunits of myosin can exist

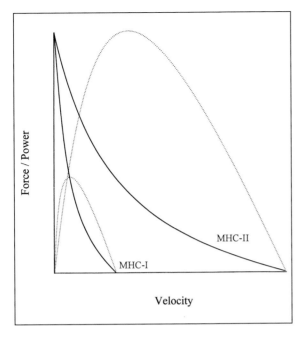

Fig. 1. Force-velocity relationship of skeletal muscle in slow (MHC-I) and fast (MHC-II) fibres. Power-velocity relationships are shown in broken lines.

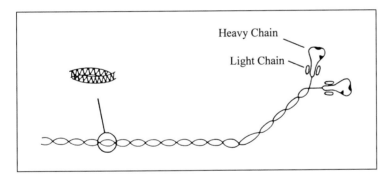

Fig. 2. Schematic diagram of a myosin molecule showing myosin heavy and light chain components.

in a number of different isoforms in mammalian muscle and these are summarised in table 1. In adult human skeletal muscle only three MHC isoforms have so far been identified, one slow (MHC-I) which seems to correspond to the β slow myosin found in cardiac muscle and two fast (MHC-IIA and MHC-IIB) isoforms. However, recent evidence has shown that the

Table 1. MHC and MLC isoforms in mammalian skeletal muscle

Gene family	Developing muscles	Fast muscles	Slow muscles
MHC	Emb-MHC Neo-MHC	MHC-IIA MHC-IIB MHC-IIX (IID)	MHC-I(β/slow)
MLC (alkali)	MLC1emb MLC3f	MLC1f MLC3f	MLC1s
MLC (regulatory)	MLC2f	MLC2f	MLC2s

From Schiaffino and Reggiani [9].

transcript for the MHC-IIB isoform in human muscle is analogous to the MHC-IIX and not the MHC-IIB isoform found in rat muscle [9, 10]. For the purposes of this review, the MHC-IIB nomenclature will remain.

The functional implications for fibres expressing different myosin iso-forms are marked. Fibres which express MHC-I isoforms exhibit V_0 values which are on average one quarter to a third slower than MHC-II (fig. 1). In fast fibres a continuum of increasing V_0 can be observed from MHC-IIA→MHC-IIX→MHC-IIB and this is associated with concomitant in-creases in power output [3]. However, within fibres which express the same MHC isoform there is considerable variability in shortening characteristics. In fast fibres of the rat this has been attributed to differences in the expression of the alkali light-chain isoforms [11]. The light chains (MLC) also show great heterogeneity. Attached to each MHC is one regulatory (DTNB extractable) isoform (MLC2s and MLC2f) and one alkali (MLC1s, MLC1f and MLC3f), with a higher proportion of MLC3f being associated with a higher V_0. In man, however, the picture is more complex as slow MLC isoforms have been shown to exist in MHC-II fibres and fast MLC isoforms in MHC-I fibres [3, 12]. In addition, individual muscle fibres may also possess more than one MHC isoform [13]. Indeed the occurrence of fibres which express only MHC-IIB isoforms are relatively rare [14], with MHC-IIB isoforms usually co-existing with MHC-IIA isoforms [14, 15]. This co-expression has a marked influence on function, with MHC-IIA/IIB fibres having a higher V_0 than fibres which express only the MHC-IIA isoform [3, 4, 16].

Myosin heavy chain adaptations

a) Fast - to - Slow Transformation

IIB → IIX → IIA → I

b) Slow - to - Fast Transformation

I → IIA → IIX (→) IIB

↓ _ _ _ _ _ _↑

Fig. 3. Order for MHC isoform transformation (a) due to chronic low frequency stimulation or mechanical loading and (b) due to intermittent high frequency stimulation (without transformation to IIB) or disuse (hind limb suspension, immobilisation, denervation, microgravity) where it has been suggested that soleus fibres in the rat possess the ability to 'jump' from expressing type I directly to IIX.

Adaptation to Usage

Animal Models

As the force-velocity properties of skeletal muscles seem to be closely regulated by the expression of the different isoforms of myosin, it seems logical to assume that if the isoforms that are expressed could be altered, then this would alter contractile function. Buller et al. [17] first demonstrated that the properties of skeletal muscle could be altered by a change in usage when in cats they re-innervated a fast muscle with the nerve normally supplied to a slow muscle. Although they did not measure MHC composition, they showed that the contractile properties of the re-innervated muscle became markedly slower, approaching that of the slow muscle. Subsequently, Salmons and Vrbová [18] extended this observation when they demonstrated in rabbit muscle that a 'fast'-to-'slow' transformation in contractile properties could be brought about by electrically stimulating the nerve with a frequency pattern which is normally delivered to a slow muscle. Since then, numerous studies have used the chronic low frequency ($\sim$10 Hz) stimulation model to induce changes in myosin expression and contractile function (fig, 3, for review, [see ref. 19]). However, it is important to emphasise at this point that the concept of 'fibre transition' is considered at the level of specific systems, as opposed to the single fibre as a single entity [20]. Indeed, the transitions of the various systems are not simultaneous, but can follow distinct time courses, with changes in the sarcoplasmic reticulum system (Ca^{2+} kinetics) and metabolism occurring earlier than the transition of myosin isoforms. Indeed, within the myosin complex itself there is evidence that the time course of MLC isoform switching may differ from that of MHC isoforms [7, 21]. Also in this regard, the time course and the extent to which fast-to-slow adaptations can be induced may vary between species, with the larger the animals the greater the affinity for conversion to slow isoforms [7].

In contrast to chronic low-frequency stimulation, less information regarding the transformation of fibres in the other direction (i.e. from slow to fast) with muscle usage is available. However, there is evidence from denervated rat soleus muscle to suggest that in contrast to continuous low-frequency stimulation, protocols which employ intermittent high-frequency (150 Hz) bursts are able to evoke a switch from the expression of slow to fast myosin isoforms with a corresponding change in contractile characteristics [22, 23] (fig. 3).

Man: A Cross-Sectional Perspective

Considerable information regarding how human skeletal muscle has adapted to usage can be obtained if one considers how muscles from different parts of the body have evolved to meet the different functional demands placed on them. A recent study [4] examined myosin expression and electrically evoked whole-muscle contractile characteristics in three muscles which differed in their functional demands. These were the plantar flexors (soleus), primarily a postural muscle group, the knee extensors (vastus lateralis) also serving a postural function, but also involved in locomotion and other dynamic activities and the elbow extensors (triceps brachii), the lightly loaded muscle of the upper arm. Clear differences in the contractile properties of three muscles were seen in vivo. The plantar flexors possessed the longest twitch time course, slowest rate of rise of tension development, highest frequency response and exhibited the greatest resistance to fatigue, while the elbow extensors exhibited the 'fastest' characteristics. These differences in contractile characteristics were coupled to the distribution of MHC isoforms in the three muscles (fig. 4). The soleus was found to be dominated by MHC-I isoforms, the vastus possessed an even distribution of MHC-I and MHC-II, with the MHC-IIA being dominant, while the triceps brachii exhibited a dominance of MHC-II isoforms with a notable proportion of MHC-IIB. A question that has remained unresolved as regards the coupling between muscle composition and contractile characteristics, is whether fibres which possess the same MHC isoforms, but which originate from different muscles, possess the same contractile properties. Using the chemically skinned single-fibre preparation, it is possible to determine V_0 in fibres extracted from a needle biopsy sample. Slack test manoeuvres to determine V_0 in single fibres from the soleus, vastus lateralis and triceps brachii muscles revealed that fibres expressing either only MHC-I or MHC-IIA isoforms exhibited a given V_0 (within a certain range, which, as described earlier, can be quite high for type II fibres), independent of the muscle of origin (table 2). Thus it seems that whole muscle contractile properties from different

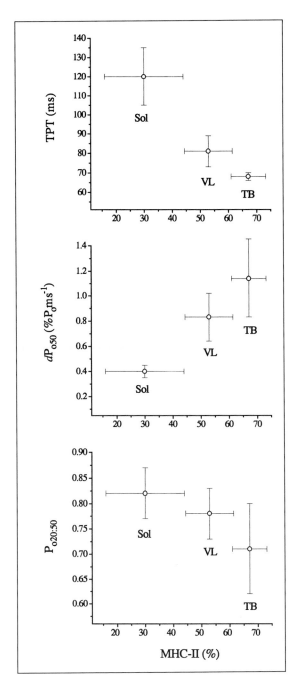

Fig. 4. Fast heavy chain (MHC-II) composition of the soleus (Sol), vastus lateralis (VL) and triceps brachii muscles (TB) in relation to twitch time to peak tension (TPT), rate of rise of tension development at 50 Hz (dP_{o50}) and the ratio of torque at 20 and 50 Hz ($P_{o20:50}$) in the plantar flexor, knee extensor and elbow extensor muscles. Data are mean ($\pm$SD) from Harridge et al. [4].

Table 2. Maximum velocity of shortening (V_0) determined at 12 °C in chemically skinned human single fibres.

	Soleus	Vastus lateralis	Triceps brachii
MHC			
Type I	0.27	0.29	0.27
SD	0.12	0.10	0.14
n	15	24	8
Type IIa	1.45	1.09	1.20
SD	0.34	0.50	0.30
n	3	10	8

Data from Harridge et al. [24].

muscles relate to the distribution in myosin isoforms and not to intrinsic differences in the properties of individual fibres from different muscles.

Another way of looking at skeletal muscle adaptation from a cross-sectional perspective is to consider athletes who excel in different physical activities. It has been known for many years that the muscles of endurance athletes show a dominance of histochemically determined slow type I fibres, while sprint and power athletes show a larger tendency towards a higher proportion of fast type II fibres [25]. The functional implications of this are shown in figure 5 which shows the force-velocity properties (in the form of torque and angular velocity) of the plantar flexors from sprint (100–400 m) and endurance (>5 km) runners. Here muscle contractions were evoked using maximal electrical stimulation at 50 Hz and a release technique to standardise muscle activation for each contraction. Even when differences in absolute strength are removed by normalising the isokinetic data to the isometric torque generated, the sprinters were able to generate higher values at all angular velocities when compared to the endurance runners—a phenomenon which was related to higher proportions of fast isomyosin in the soleus and gastrocnemius muscles in these athletes [26, 27].

Man: A Longitudinal Perspective

The extent to which these differences between athletes result from genetic predisposition or from years of adaptation to training is unclear. Over recent years numerous training studies have been performed which have examined the effects of different training regimes on the composition of human muscle

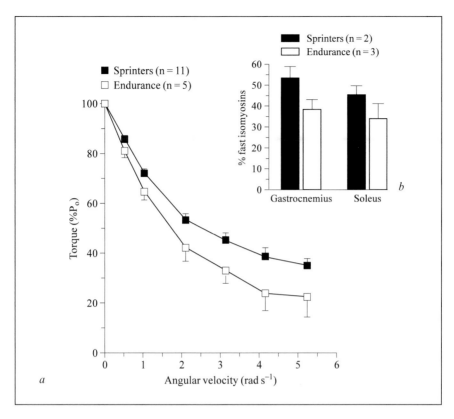

Fig. 5. a Torque-angular velocity data from the plantar flexors obtained from stimulated release contractions at 50 Hz. *b* Fast isomyosin composition of the soleus and gastrocnemius of sprint and endurance athletes. Adapted from Harridge et al. [26] and Harridge [27].

(table 3). However, few consistent changes have been observed as regards the distribution of the major fibre types with either power or endurance-based training protocols. In contrast to the marked changes that have been observed during chronic stimulation, less obvious changes are seen. However, it must be remembered that these changes in animal muscle have occurred as a result of non-physiological stimuli for up to 12–24 h per day and less evidence of changes in the major fibre types as a result of physiological training is available [19]. Furthermore, in man physical training regimes can only be superimposed on the daily activities of the individual, which must involve delivering conflicting signals to the muscle. For example sprint training information, i.e. high-frequency intermittent bursts, can only be superimposed on the more chronic low-frequency stimulation that will occur during more prolonged

Table 3. Fibre composition changes (myosin ATPase histochemistry of the vastus lateralis) in response to high-intensity (sprint/power)-based and low-intensity (endurance)-based training regimes in man.

Reference	Duration of bout	Duration of training		Type, %		
				I	IIA	IIB
High intensity						
Simoneau et al. [28]	15–90 s	(4–5)	15 wks	↑	↔	↓
Jansson et al. [29]	30 s	(2–3)	4–6 wks	↓	↑	↔
Jacobs et al. [30]	15–30 s	(2–3)	6 wks	↘	↑	↔
Esbjörnsson et al. [31]	10 s	(3)	6 wks	↓	↑	↓
Linossier et al. [32]	5 s	(4)	7 wks	↑	↔	↓
Staron et al. [33] (strength)	3 × 6–12 s (70–85%)	(2)	6–13 wks	↔	↑	↓
Adams et al. [34] (strength)	3 × 6–12 s (70–85%)	(2)	19 wks	↔	↗	↓
Cadefeau et al. [35]	–		8 months	↑	↓	↓
Low intensity						
Andersen and Henriksson [36]	30 min	(4)	8 wks	↔	↑	↓
Howald et al. [37]	30 min	(5)	6 wks	↑	↗	↓
Bauman et al. [38]	30 min	(5)	8 wks	↔	↑	↓
Ingjer [39] (cross-country skiing)	45 min	(3)	24 wks	↔	↑	↓

Training was in the form of cycling unless stated otherwise. Training days per week indicated in parenthesis.

postural activities. In addition, most human training studies are only performed for a limited period of time, both in terms of the total time spent each day and the total number of days trained. A further reason for the lack of changes in muscle composition with training in humans may also relate to the traditional histochemical (myosin ATPase) method of determining fibre composition, which may not be sensitive enough to reveal co-expression of MHC isoforms in individual fibres. Indeed, both strength [40] and endurance [41] athletes have been shown to have a greater number of fibres which co-express more than one MHC isoform.

The most common feature of both endurance and sprint-based training regimes seems to be a loss of type IIB fibres. It seems that the majority of MHC-IIB isoforms are co-expressed with MHC-IIA isoforms. However, the consistency with which the IIB fibres are reduced with training suggests that this isoform is highly sensitive to increased usage. It has been suggested that the MHC-IIB (or IIX) is the default gene [6, 34] which transforms into MHC-IIA with increases in any form of usage. Indeed in agreement with this argument, a very recent study [41] reported that even a sprint training protocol which employed repeated sprints of extremely short duration (3 s) resulted in a decline in MHC-IIB isoform composition. Interestingly, in that study V_0 of fibres expressing only MHC-I or MHC-IIA isoforms were unaltered with training. This finding is in contrast to an earlier study [43] which reported that single-fibre V_0 in MHC-II fibres from the deltoid muscle was reduced after intense swim training. However, no differentiation was made between MHC-IIA and MHC-IIB isoforms in the swim training study. As a number of those fibres were likely to express MHC-IIB isoforms, which were likely to be reduced with training, V_0 after training was probably a reflection of the V_0 of MHC-IIA fibres.

A recent sprint training study [15] observed that the number of fibres expressing only the MHC-IIA isoform was increased after training. This appeared to be at the expense of both MHC-IIB and MHC-I isoforms. This prompted the suggestion that a bidirectional change in MHC isoform expression (I→IIA←IIB) was possible in human fibres with this type of training.

Adaptation to Disuse

As well as an increase, or change, in the type of muscle usage, marked alterations in the pattern of myosin isoform expression may result from disuse. For example, following 4 weeks of hind limb suspension of the rat, the amount of MHC-I expressed in the soleus was shown to be markedly reduced, whilst MHC-II isoforms [44], were shown to increase. A similar phenomenon has recently been reported in spinal-cord-transected rats [45], where a down-regulation of slow isoforms and an up-regulation of fast isoforms seemed to proceed in the same direction as that described for slow to fast transformations as a result of intermittent high-frequency stimulation (fig. 3). The appearance of MHC-IIB isoforms appears to be unique with regard to immobilisation or denervation. In that study, there was also evidence to suggest that some fibres possess the ability to 'jump' from expressing MHC-I to MHC-IIX without expressing the MHC-IIA isoform [45]. In addition, the regulation of isoform expression does not seem to depend solely on the level of neural input, but also on mechanical strain. In a recent study, immobilization of the fast-twitch rabbit tibialis anterior muscle in a stretched position was shown to exhibit isoform switching in a fast-to-slow direction [6].

In man, a reduction in the proportion of histochemically identified type I fibres has been shown in the vastus lateralis following 5 weeks of cast immobilisation following surgery [46]. However, in the same muscle, 4 weeks of unloading [47] or 30 days of tilted bed-rest [48] did not result in any change in the relative proportion of the different fibre types. In contrast, 11 days of microgravity (space flight) seemed to be sufficient to result in a decrease in the proportion of fibres expressing MHC-I isoforms, although no increase in the number of fibres expressing MHC-IIB was observed [49]. In patients with spinal cord injuries where permanent muscular paralysis results, a very pronounced reduction in histochemically identified type I fibres [50–52] and MHC-I isoforms [53] is observed. This is accompanied by a marked increase in the proportion of type IIB fibres and the number of fibres expressing only MHC-IIB isoforms. Recent evidence suggests, however, that even after long-term disuse, human skeletal muscle is capable of exhibiting plasticity. Chronic stimulation (20 Hz) of the tibialis anterior for 24 weeks resulted in a marked shift away from type IIB fibres with an increase in type I fibres [51]. In a very recent study, 1 year of electrically evoked cycle training, performed for just 30 min repeated three times per week, evoked a marked decrease in the number fibres expressing MHC-IIB and a dramatic increase in the number of fibres expressing the MHC-IIA isoform. There was, however, no significant increase in the number of fibres expressing MHC I [53].

References

1   Reiser PJ, Moss RL, Giulian GG, Greaser ML: Shortening velocity in single fibres from adult rabbit soleus muscles is correlated with myosin heavy chain composition. J Biol Chem 1985;260: 9077–9080.
2   Bottinelli R, Schiaffino S, Reggiani C: Force-velocity relations and myosin heavy chain isoform compositions of skinned fibres from rat skeletal muscle. J Physiol (Lond) 1991;437:655–672.
3   Larsson L, Moss RL: Maximum velocity of shortening in relation to myosin isoform composition in single fibres from human skeletal muscles. J Physiol (Lond) 1993;472:595–614.
4   Harridge SDR, Bottinelli R, Reggiani C, Esbjörnsson M, Cancepari M, Pellegrino M, Saltin B: Whole muscle and single fibre contractile characteristics in relation to myosin isoform expression in man, submitted.
5   Hill AV: The design of muscle. Br Med Bul 1956;12:165–166.
6   Goldspink G, Scutt A, Martindale J, Jaenicke T, Turay L, Gerlach GF: Stretch and force generation induce rapid hypertrophy and myosin isoform gene switching in adult skeletal muscle. Biochem Soc Trans 1991;19:368–373.
7   Booth F, Thomason DB: Molecular and cellular adaptation of muscle in response to exercise: Perspectives of various models. Physiol Rev 71:541–585.
8   Smerdu V, Karsch-Mizrachi I, Campione M, Leinwand L, Schaffino S: Type IIx myosin heavy chain transcripts are expressed in type IIb fibres of human skeletal muscle. Am J Physiol 1994;267: C1723–C1728.
9   Schiaffino S, Reggiani C: Myosin isoforms in mammalian skeletal muscle. J Appl Physiol 1994;7: 493–501.

10 Ennion S, Sant'ana Pereira JAA, Sargeant AJ, Young A, Goldspink G: Characterization of human skeletal muscle fibres according to the myosin heavy chains they express. J Muscle Res Cell Motil 1995;16:35–43.

11 Bottinelli R, Betto R, Schiaffino, S, Reggiani C: Unloaded shortening velocity and myosin heavy and alkali light chain isoform composition in rat skeletal muscle fibres. J Physiol (Lond) 1994;478: 341–349.

12 Billeter R, Heizmann CW, Howald H, Jenny E: Analysis of myosin light and heavy chain types in single human skeletal muscle fibres. Eur J Biochem 1981;116:389–395.

13 Biral D, Betto R, Danieli-Betto D, Salviati G, Myosin heavy chain composition of single fibres from normal human muscle, Biochem J 1988;250:307–308.

14 Klitgaard H, Zhou M, Schiaffino S, Betto R, Salviati G, Saltin B: Ageing alters the myosin heavy chain composition of single fibres from human skeletal muscle. Acta Physiol Scand 1990;140:55–62.

15 Andersen JL, Klitgaard H, Saltin B: Myosin heavy chain isoforms in single fibres from m.vastus lateralis of sprinters: Influence of training intensity. Acta Physiol Scand 1993;151:135–142.

16 Bottinelli R, Betto R, Schiaffino S, Reggiani C: Maximum shortening velocity and coexistence of myosin heavy chain isoforms in single skinned fast fibres of rat skeletal muscle. J Muscle Res Cell Motil 1994;15:413–419.

17 Buller AJ, Eccles JC, Eccles RM: Interactions between motoneurones and muscles in respect of the characteristic speeds of their responses. J Physiol (Lond) 1960;150:417–439.

18 Salmons S, Vrbová G: The influence of activity on some contractile characteristics of mammalian fast and slow muscles. J Physiol (Lond) 1969;210:535–549.

19 Pette D, Vrbová G: Adaptation of mammalian skeletal muscle fibers to chronic electrical stimulation. Rev Physiol Biochem Pharmacol 1992;120:115–202.

20 Green HJ, Klug GA, Reichmann H, Seedorf U, Wieher W, Pette D: Exercise-induced fibre transitions with regard to myosin, paravalbumin, and sarcoplasmic reticulum in muscles of the rat. Pflügers Arch 1984;400:432–438.

21 Heilig A, Pette D: Changes in transcriptional activity of chronically stimulated fast twitch muscle. FEBS Lett 1983;151:211–214.

22 Ausoni S, Gorza L, Schiaffino S, Gunderson K, Lomo T: Myosin heavy chain isoforms in stimulated fast and slow rat muscles. J Neurol Sci 1990;10:153–160.

23 Gorza L, Gundersen K, Lømo T, Schiaffino S, Westgaard RH: Slow-to-fast transformation of denervated soleus muscles by chronic high frequency stimulation in the rat. J Physiol (Lond) 1988; 402:627–649.

24 Harridge SDR, Bottinelli R, Reggiani C, Pellegrino MA, Canepari M, Saltin B: Similar maximum velocity of shortening in single fibres expressing the same myosin heavy chain, but from different human skeletal muscles. J Physiol (Lond) (abstract) 487P.152P.

25 Saltin B, Gollnick PD: Skeletal muscle adaptability, significance for metabolism and performance; in Handbook of Physiology. Section 10: Skeletal Muscle. Bethesda/Baltimore, American Physiological Society Williams & Wilkins, 1983, pp 555–663.

26 Harridge SDR, White MJ, Carrington CA, Goodman M, Cummins P: Electrically evoked torque-velocity characteristics and isomyosin composition of the triceps surae in young and elderly men. Acta Physiol Scand 1995;154:469–477.

27 Harridge SDR: Determinants of the torque-velocity relationship of the human triceps surae; PhD thesis, Birmingham, 1993.

28 Simoneau J-A, Lortie G, Boulay MR, Marcotte M, Thibault M-C, Bouchard C: Human skeletal muscle fiber type alteration with high-intensity intermittent training. Eur J Appl Physiol 1985;54:250–253.

29 Jansson E, Esbjörnsson M, Holm I, Jacobs I: Increase in the proportion of fast-twitch muscle fibres by sprint training in males. Acta Physiol Scand 1990;140:359–363.

30 Jacobs I, Esbjörnsson M, Sylvén C, Holm I, Jansson E: Sprint training effects on muscle myoglobin, enzymes, fiber types, and blood lactate. Med Sci Sport Exerc 1987;19:368–374.

31 Esbjörnsson M, Hellsten-Westing Y, Balsom PD, Sjödin B, Jansson, E, Muscle fibre type changes with sprint training: Effect of training pattern. Acta Physiol Scand 1993;149:245–246.

32 Linossier M-T, Denis C, Dormois D, Geyssant A, Lacour JR: Ergometric and metabolic adaptation to a 5-s spring training programme. Eur J Appl Physiol 1993;67:408–414.

33 Staron, RS, Malicky, ES, Leonardi MJ, Falkel JE, Hagerman FC, Dudley GA: Muscle hypertrophy and fast fibre type conversions in heavy resistance-trained women. Eur J Appl Physiol 1989;61: 71–79.

34 Adams GR, Hather BM, Balwin KM, Dudley GA: Skeletal muscle myosin heavy chain composition and resistance training. J Appl Physiol 1993;74:911–915.

35 Cadefau J, Casademonte J, Grau JM, Fernández J, Balaguer A, Vernet M, Cussó, R Urbano-Márquez A: Biochemical and histochemical adaptation to sprint training in young athletes. Acta Physiol Scand 1990;140:341–351.

36 Andersen P, Henriksson J: Training induced changes in the subgroups of human type II skeletal muscle fibres. Acta Physiol Scand 1975;99:123–125.

37 Howald HH, Hoppeler H, Classen H, Mathieu O, Straub R: Influences of endurance training on the ultra-structural comparison of the different muscle fibre types in humans. Pflügers Arch 1985; 403:369–376.

38 Baumann H, Jäggi M, Howald H, Schaub MC: Exercise training induces transitions of myosin isoform subunits with histochemically typed human muscle fibres. Pflügers Arch 1987;409:349–360.

39 Ingjer F: Effects of endurance training on muscle fibre ATPase activity, capillary supply and mitochondrial content in man. J Physiol (Lond) 1979;294:419–432.

40 Klitgaard H, Bergman O, Betto R, Salviati G, Schiaffino S, Clausen T, Saltin B: Co-existence of myosin heavy chain I and IIa isoforms in human skeletal muscle fibres with endurance training. Pflügers Arch 1990;416:471–472.

41 Klitgaard, Zhou M, Richter EA: Myosin heavy chain composition of single fibres from m. biceps brachii of male body builders. Acta Physiol Scand 1990;140:175–180.

42 Bottinelli R, Harridge SDR, Canepari M, Reggiani C, Saltin B: Effect of training on myosin heavy chain isoform distribution and maximum shortening velocity of single human skeletal muscle fibres (abstract). Pflügers Arch, in press.

43 Fitts RH, Costill DA, Gardetto PR: Effect of swim training on human muscle fibre function. J Appl Physiol 1989;242:65–73.

44 Thomason DB, Herrick RE, Surdyka D, Baldwin KM: Time course of soleus muscle myosin expression during hindlimb suspension and recovery. J Appl Physiol 1987;63:130–137.

45 Talmadge RJ, Roy RR, Edgerton VR: Prominence of myosin heavy chain hybrid fibers in soleus muscle of spinal chord transected rats. J Appl Physiol 1995;78:1256–1265.

46 Häggmark T, Jansson E, Eriksson E: Fiber type area and metabolic potential of the thigh muscle in man after knee surgery and immobilization. Int J Sports Med 1981;2:12–17.

47 Berg HE, Dudley GA, Hather B, Tesch P: Work capacity and metabolic and morphological characteristics of the human quadriceps muscle in response to unloading. Clin Physiol 1993;13:337–347.

48 Hikida RS, Gollnick PD, Dudley GA, Convertino VA, Buchanan P: Structural and metabolic characteristics of human skeletal muscle following 30 days of simulated microgravity. Aviat Space Environ Med 1989;60:664–670.

49 Zhou M-Y, Klitgaard H, Saltin B, Roy RR, Edgerton VR, Gollnick PD: Myosin heavy chain isoforms of human muscle after short-term spaceflight. J Appl Physiol 1995;78:1740–1744.

50 Grimby G, Broberg C, Krotkiewska I, Krotiewski M: Muscle fiber composition in patients with traumatic lesion. Scand J Rehabil Med 1976;8:37–42.

51 Martin TP, Stein R, Hoeppner PH, Reid DC: Influence of electrical stimulation on the morphological and metabolic properties of paralyzed muscle. J Appl Physiol 1992;72:1401–1406.

52 Round JM, Barr FMD, Moffat, B, Jones DA: Fibre areas and histochemical fibre types in the quadriceps muscle of paraplegic subjects. J Neurol Sci 1993;116:207–211.

53 Andersen JL, Mohr T, Biering-Sørenson F, Galbo H, Kjær M: Myosin heavy chain isoform transformation in single fibres from m. vastus lateralis in spinal cord injured individuals: Effects of long terms functional electrical stimulation (FES). Pflügers Arch, in press.

Dr. Stephen D.R. Harridge, Copenhagen Muscle Research Centre, Rigshospitalet, Section 7652, DK–2200 Copenhagen (Denmark)

Marconnet P, Saltin B, Komi P, Poortmans J (eds): Human Muscular Function
during Dynamic Exercise. Med Sport Sci. Basel, Karger, 1996, vol 41, pp 95–101

....
Adaptations of the Antioxidant Defence Systems to Chronic Exercises

Garry G. Duthie

Rowett Research Institute, Bucksburn, Aberdeen, UK

Regular exercise is regarded as being beneficial to health. However, acute exercise by untrained individuals can produce muscle soreness and injury [1]. The mechanisms underlying exercise-induced muscle damage are unclear but have been partly ascribed to endogenously produced free radicals. Such damage does not occur to the same extent in trained individuals who undergo chronic exercise exposure [2]. The aim of this paper is to discuss whether the amelioration of the adverse effects of exercise by training reflects adaptive responses by the cellular antioxidant defence mechanisms.

Reactive Oxygen Species

During oxidative phosphorylation, superoxide radicals (O_2^-) are produced in mitochondria when single electrons react with molecular oxygen. During basal metabolism, 1–4% of O_2^- originating in the mitochondria may leak into the cytosol where iron or copper catalysis can promote the formation of highly reactive hydroxyl ($OH°$) radicals or a similar species with comparable activity. Moreover, in the respiratory chain during univalent reduction of oxygen, a semiquinone radical in the presence of hydrogen peroxide and high hydrogen ion concentration may also propagate the formation of $OH°$. These reactive oxygen species (ROS) can abstract hydrogen atoms from a wide range of biomolecules including the polyunsaturated fatty acids of cell and organelle membranes. Resulting oxidation of the lipid and protein components of biological membranes may result in loss of membrane integrity and tissue damage. Moreover, ROS can also disrupt cellular calcium (Ca^{2+}) homeostasis by inactivation of regulatory mechanisms such as Ca^{2+}-ATPase pumps, Na^+-Ca^{2+}

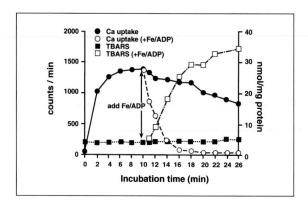

Fig. 1. Addition of iron/ADP to generate $OH°$-type radicals causes rapid loss of Ca^{2+} from hepatic microsomes as indicated by the open circles. Closed circles indicate addition of saline as comparative control. Addition of iron/ADP results in the formation of indices of lipid peroxidation (open squares) estimated as thiobarbituric acid-reactive substances (TBARS). Addition of saline does not promote the formation of thiobarbituric-acid-reactive substances.

exchange mechanisms and the voltage-sensitive ryanodine receptor. The subsequent loss of control of the asymmetric movements of Ca^{2+} across the cellular membranes can then precipitate the death of the cell by activation of potentially destructive biochemical pathways involving phospholipase A_2, neutral proteases and lysosomal acid hydrolases [3]. For example, generation of ROS markedly affects $^{45}Ca^{2+}$ uptake by the hepatic microsomal Ca^{2+}-ATPase pump (fig. 1). Moreover, the ROS-induced efflux of Ca^{2+} is associated with an increase in thiobarbituric-acid-reactive substances suggesting damage to the lipid components of the microsomal membrane.

Antioxidant Defence Systems

Cells are protected from the potentially injurious effects of free radicals by antioxidant defence systems. Antioxidants are substances which, when present at much lower concentrations than an oxidisable substrate, significantly delay or prevent its oxidation. Endogenous antioxidants such as glutathione and ubiquinone are synthesised by cells whereas other essential antioxidants have to be taken up from the diet. Vitamin E is a major lipid-soluble antioxidant which breaks the chain of free-radical-mediated lipid peroxidation of polyunsaturated fatty acids in cell membranes. β-Carotene and other carotenoids may have a similar function particularly in tissues with a low partial pressure

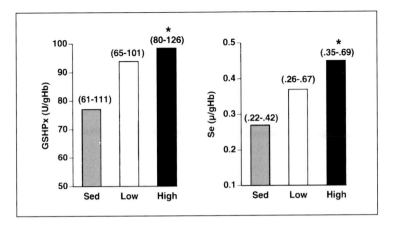

Fig. 2. Activities of glutathione peroxidase (GSHPx) and concentrations of selenium (Se), the cofactor of the antioxidant enzyme, in subjects who had primarily sedentary lifestyles (Sed, n = 6) or had been undertaking either low (16–43 km, n = 6) or high (80–147 km, n = 6) weekly running training for at least 2 years.

of oxygen. Vitamin C scavenges free radicals in the water-soluble compartment of the cell and may regenerate vitamin E. In addition, several antioxidant enzymes such as glutathione peroxidase, catalase and superoxide dismutase remove the toxic intermediates produced on oxidation of biological material. These enzymes require metal cofactors (selenium for glutathione peroxidase, iron for catalase, copper, zinc and manganese for superoxide dismutase) [4].

Adaptations of Antioxidant Defence Systems

Aerobic metabolic rate increases up to 10-fold during physical exercise enhancing leakage of O_2^- from the mitochondria to the cytosol. Detection of free radical signals and elevated indices of lipid peroxidation in plasma and tissues of untrained humans and animals following bouts of acute activity suggests that exercise-induced rises in ROS exceed the protective capacity of the antioxidant defence system [5–8]. However, upregulation of antioxidant defences occurs in response to sustained oxidative loads arising from genetic disorders, nutritional antioxidant deficiencies and smoking: these effects may be mediated directly by ROS or indirectly by hormones, cytokines and the metal cofactors which impose pre- and post-translational control over the genetic expression of antioxidant enzymes. Therefore, similar adaptations are likely in response to sustained ROS production by chronic exercise.

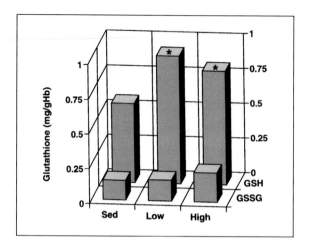

Fig. 3. Values for erythrocyte reduced and oxidised glutathione (GSH and GSSG, respectively) in subjects who had primarily sedentary lifestyles (Sed, n = 6) or had been undertaking either low (16–43 km, n = 6) or high (80–147 km, n = 6) weekly running training for at least 2 years.

For example, there are marked differences in blood antioxidant concentrations and antioxidant enzyme activities when subjects with sedentary lifestyle are compared with those who train regularly. Erythrocyte glutathione peroxidase (fig. 2) and catalase activities rise in proportion to weekly training distance although superoxide dismutase activity remains unaltered [9]. Similarly, exercise training of rats causes proportionate enhancement of muscle mitochondrial and cytosolic glutathione peroxidase [10], and catalase is reported to increase in human skeletal muscle after training [11]. These exercise-induced changes in muscle antioxidant enzymes may be muscle specific. For example, following treadwheel training of female rats at three levels of exercise intensity for 10 weeks, glutathione peroxidase activity increased only in red gastrocnemius muscle whereas superoxide dismutase activity was elevated in soleus [12]. Training also induces marked increases in erythrocyte GSH concentrations (fig. 3) which in addition to enhancing the antioxidant capacity of the red cell, may contribute to vitamin E recycling and to the restoration of the activity of thiol-dependent enzymes after exercise-induced inactivation. The concentration of GSH in plasma may also depend on the training status of the exercising subject. For example, increased plasma GSH in trained subjects may arise because adapted skeletal muscle may deliver GSH into the circulation. Decreased plasma GSH following exercise by untrained individuals may reflect increased GSH consumption by muscle resulting in decreased export of GSH to plasma [13].

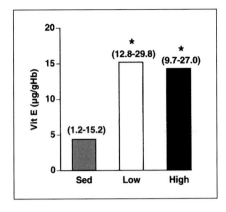

Fig. 4. Concentrations of vitamin E in erythrocytes of subjects who had primarily sedentary lifestyles (Sed, n = 6) or had been undertaking either low (16–43 km, n = 6) or high (80–147 km, n = 6) weekly running training for at least 2 years.

Chronic exercise is also associated with alterations in blood antioxidant vitamin concentrations which cannot be ascribed solely to fluid shifts from plasma to tissues. For example, increases in plasma vitamin C concentrations in athletes have been ascribed to the efflux of ascorbate from the adrenal gland associated with post-exercise increases in plasma cortisol [14]. Similarly, increases in erythrocyte vitamin E content also occurs after prolonged intensive exercise which may indicate mobilisation of the antioxidant from tissues and plasma [15].

Although changes in concentrations of antioxidants and activities of antioxidant enzymes may be in response to chronic exercise, they may also be attributed in part to the effects of altered food intakes. Daily energy intake is strongly related to the amount of physical training and therefore increased antioxidant status may reflect greater intakes of foods containing antioxidant nutrients and the metal cofactors for antioxidant enzymes. Consequently, observed increase in erythrocyte vitamin E concentration of trained athletes (fig. 4) may reflect in part greater consumption of foods containing this important antioxidant vitamin.

Antioxidant Supplementation

Increases in plasma and tissue antioxidant concentrations and antioxidant enzyme activities in trained athletes compared with sedentary individuals indicate adaptive upregulation of the antioxidant defence system. This is likely to be a response to enhanced, persistent oxidative loads arising from sustained exercise. However, as increased blood oxidised glutathione concentrations and creatine kinase activities occur in dedicated athletes who run 80–147 km/week [9], such adaptation may be insufficient to completely protect individuals who train extensively. Consequently, numerous studies have assessed the benefits of augmenting the antioxidant defence system by supplementation with antioxidants such as vitamin E [16–19]. Despite differences in exercise protocols, supplementation periods and training status of subjects, most studies with human subjects indicate that increased vitamin E intakes lower indices of lipid peroxidation following exercise when compared with subjects on placebo. As elevated indices of lipid peroxidation have been implicated in the pathogenesis of many diseases [20], individuals who train excessively should consider increasing their intakes of nutritional antioxidants. However, whether optimum intakes can be achieved by dietary means or require recourse to supplements is not clear.

Conclusion

Reactive oxygen species such as superoxide are produced as a by-product of metabolism. Basal aerobic metabolic rate may increase 10-fold during physical exercise and result in enhanced leakage of superoxide from mitochondria to the cytosol. In untrained individuals, the rise in oxygen-derived free radical concentrations may exceed the protective capacity of the antioxidant defence system and result in tissue damage as indicated by perturbations in calcium homeostasis, muscle soreness and increased plasma indices of lipid peroxidation and creatine kinase activities. Chronic exercise results in increased concentrations of antioxidant vitamins and enhanced activities of antioxidant enzymes in blood and tissues suggesting adaptive responses of the antioxidant defence system to a sustained free-radical load. For example, regular running causes increased red cell vitamin E and glutathione concentrations and enhanced glutathione peroxidase and catalase activities which are reflected by decreases in plasma indices of lipid peroxidation. Nevertheless, such compensation for the increased free-radical load appears insufficient to ameliorate muscle damage in individuals who regularly run in excess of 100 km/week, possibly indicating an increased requirement for antioxidants such as vitamin E.

Acknowlegements

Funding is appreciated from the Scottish Office Agriculture and Fisheries Department (SOAFD), BASF Germany, and the Ministry of Agriculture, Fisheries and Food, UK.

References

1 Armstrong RB, Warren GL, Warren JA: Mechanisms of exercise-induced muscle fibre injury. Sports Med 1991;12:184–207.
2 Jenkins R: Free radical chemistry: Relationship to exercise. Sports Med 1988;5:156–170.
3 Duthie GG, Arthur JR: Free radicals and calcium homeostasis: Relevance to malignant hyperthermia. Free Radic Biol Med 1993;14:435–442.
4 Duthie GG: Vitamin E and antioxidants. Chem Ind 1992;16:598–601.
5 Davies KJA, Quintanilha AT, Brooks GA, Packer L: Free radicals and tissue damage produced by exercise. Biochem Biophys Res Commun 1982;107:1198–1205.
6 Lovlin R, Cottle W, Pyke I, Kavanagh M, Belcastro AN: Are indices of free radical damage related to exercise intensity? Eur J Appl Physiol 1987;56:313–316.
7 Dillard CJ, Litov RE, Savin WM, Dumelin EE, Tappel AL: Effects of exercise, vitamin E, and ozone on pulmonary function and lipid peroxidation. J Appl Physiol 1987;45:927–932.
8 Maughan RJ, Donnelly AE, Gleeson M, Whiting PH, Walker KA, Clough PJ: Delayed-onset muscle damage and lipid peroxidation in man after a downhill run. Muscle Nerve 1989;12:332–336.
9 Robertson JD, Maughan RJ, Duthie GG, Morrice PC: Increased blood antioxidant systems of runners in response to training load. Clin Sci 1991;80:611–618.
10 Ji LL, Stratman FW, Lardy HA: Antioxidant enzyme systems in rat liver and muscle. Archiv Biochem Biophys 1988;263:150–160.
11 Jenkins RR, Friendland R, Howard H: The relationship of oxygen uptake to superoxide dismutase and catalase activity in human muscle. Int J Sports Med 1984;5:11–14.
12 Powers SK, Criswell D, Lawler J, Ji LL, Martin D, Herb RA, Dudley G: Influence of exercise and fiber type on antioxidant enzyme activity in rat skeletal muscle. Am J Physiol 1994;266:R375–R380.
13 Kretzschmar M, Muller D: Aging, training and exercise. A review of effects on plasma glutathione and lipid peroxides. Sports Med 1993;15:196–209.
14 Gleeson M, Robertson JD, Maughan RJ: Influence of exercise on ascorbic acid status in man. Clin Sci 1987;73:501–505.
15 Duthie GG, Robertson JR, Maughan RJ, Morrice PC: Blood antioxidant status and erythrocyte lipid peroxidation following distance running. Arch Biochem Biophys 1990;262:78–83.
16 Dillard CJ, Litov RE, Savin WM, Dumelin EE, Tappel AL: Effects of exercise, vitamin E, and ozone on pulmonary function and lipid peroxidation. J Appl Physiol 1978;45:927–932.
17 Meydani M, Evans WJ, Handelman G, Biddle L, Fielding RA, Meydani SN, Burrill J, Fiatarone MA, Blumberg JB, Cannon JG: Protective effect of vitamin E on exercise-induced oxidative damage in young and older adults. Am J Physiol 1993;264:R992–R998.
18 Simon-Schnass I, Pabst H: Influence of vitamin E on physical performance. Int J Vitam Nutr Res 1988;58:49–54.
19 Sumida S, Tanaka K, Kitao H, Nakadomo F: Exercise-induced lipid peroxidation and leakage of enzymes before and after vitamin E supplementation. Int J Biochem 1989;21:835–838.
20 Duthie GG: Lipid peroxidation. Eur J Clin Nutr 1993;47:759–764.

Dr. Garry Duthie, Principal Research Scientist. The Rowett Research Institute, Greenburn Road, Bucksburn, Aberdeen, AB2 9SB (UK)

Marconnet P, Saltin B, Komi P, Poortmans J (eds): Human Muscular Function during Dynamic Exercise. Med Sport Sci. Basel, Karger, 1996, vol 41, pp 102–120

··

Adenine Nucleotide Metabolism – A Role in Free Radical Generation and Protection?

Ylva Hellsten

Copenhagen Muscle Research Centre, August Krogh Institute, Copenhagen, Denmark

Introduction

In skeletal muscle, adenine nucleotides play a pivotal role in the transfer of chemical energy, obtained from aerobic and anaerobic energy processes, to mechanical energy used for contraction. During intensive exercise, when the energy utilization is very rapid, degradation of adenine nucleotides is essential in order to maintain a high energy charge and, thus, proper energy delivery. Recently, adenine nucleotide metabolism during intense exercise has been found to be involved in a rather different area, namely in free-radical generation and protection. In the final part of the adenine nucleotide degradation pathway in which nucleotides are degraded to purines, a free-radical-generating enzyme is involved: xanthine oxidase. This enzyme can exist in two forms, a dehydrogenase and an oxidase form and although both forms of the enzyme catalyse the same two reactions, oxidation of hypoxanthine to xanthine and oxidation of xanthine to uric acid, the electron acceptor specificity is different for the two forms. In the xanthine-dehydrogenase-catalysed reaction, nicotine amide dinucleotide (NAD^+) is utilized as the sole electron acceptor whereas xanthine oxidase utilises molecular oxygen. The univalent reduction of oxygen leads to the formation of superoxide radicals.

$$\text{Hypoxanthine} + NAD^+ + H_2O \quad \overset{\text{xanthine}}{\underset{}{\Rightarrow}} \quad \text{xanthine} + NADH + H^+ \tag{1}$$

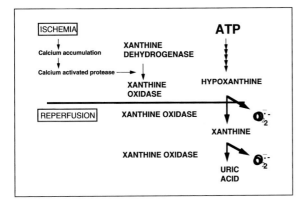

Fig. 1. Schematic representation of free radical generation via xanthine oxidase in the ischaemia/reperfusion model proposed by Granger [10] and McCord [58]. See text for details.

$$\text{Hypoxanthine} + O_2 + H_2O \quad \overset{\text{xanthine oxidase}}{\Rightarrow} \quad \text{xanthine} + O_2^{-} + H^{+} \tag{2}$$

In normal tissue, between 70 and 90% of the total enzyme activity exists in the dehydrogenase form [1–3] but under certain conditions, a conversion from the dehydrogenase to the oxidase form can occur [4, 5]. Based on the above properties, xanthine oxidase has been suggested to be one of the potential sources of oxygen radicals in the muscle tissue during exercise when the level of metabolic stress is high [6]. The present chapter will discuss the potential of free-radical generation via xanthine oxidase[1] during exercise based on the indirect evidence that exists of such an event.

There is an alternative possibility of an involvement of xanthine oxidase in excercise: the secondary inflammatory phase that may occur following exercise-induced muscle damage [7]. The theory of a role for xanthine in the immunological system has become increasingly widespread in the clinical area as numerous studies have documented an interaction between xanthine oxidase and immunoparticipating mediators and cells [8–10]. Among other effects, several immunomodulators have been shown to induce a conversion of xanthine dehydrogenase to its oxidase form [11, 12]. Findings with regard to the participation of xanthine oxidase in immunological events and the possible implications for the exercise situation will be discussed.

[1] The enzyme will be referred to as xanthine oxidase, except when specifically referring to the dehydrogenase form.

Somewhat paradoxical, free-radical generation via the xanthine oxidase reaction is paralleled by the formation of a free-radical scavenger. Uric acid, the second product in the xanthine oxidase reaction, has been found in vitro and, to some extent, in vivo to be an efficient scavenger of free radicals, including the highly reactive hydroxyl radical [13–15]. Uric acid exists in high concentrations in plasma of most mammals including man and it has been suggested that the plasma uric acid concentration of different animals is in fact correlated to longevity. Recent studies demonstrate that uric acid may be an important free-radical scavenger in muscle during exercise [16]. An overview will be given of the findings with regard to uric acid as a scavenger of radicals during various experimental conditions, including exercise.

Free-Radical Generation via Xanthine Oxidase in Muscle during Exercise

A group of researchers including Granger et al. [17] and McCord [18] first described the theory of harmful free radicals being formed via xanthine oxidase during conditions of metabolic stress in tissue, in their case represented by ischemia followed by reperfusion. These investigators demonstrated that the in vitro conversion of xanthine dehydrogenase to xanthine oxidase, which had been observed by Della Corte and Stirpe [4], also occurred in situ [18] and in vivo [17] during ischaemia. According to their theory, ischaemia leads to a degradation of adenine nucleotides and a consequent impairment of the ATP-dependent calcium pumps. The rise in intracellular calcium causes the activation of calcium-dependent proteases which act on xanthine dehydro-genase leading to the conversion to the oxidase form (fig. 1). When the tissue is reperfused with blood, oxygen and hypoxanthine formed during the ischaemic phase becomes available for the xanthine oxidase reaction, whereby superoxide radicals are formed (fig. 1).

Although the muscle does not suffer from total hypoxia during dynamic exercise, the metabolic conditions of skeletal muscle during intense exercise appear to resemble those of ischaemic tissue in several aspects. In the following sections, the requirements for generation of free radicals via xanthine oxidase in conjunction with exercise in humans will be reviewed: (1) presence of xanthine oxidase in human skeletal muscle tissue; (2) conversion from the dehydrogenase to the oxidase form; (3) presence of hypoxanthine, or xanthine, the substrates of xanthine oxidase. In the final section indications of free-radical generation via xanthine oxidase and evidence for free-radical formation in human skeletal muscle during intense exercise will be presented [4].

Table 1. Xanthine dehydrogenase/oxidase activities in human tissues

Tissue	Xanthine oxidase activity nmol $\cdot$ min^{-1} $\cdot$ g^{-1} protein	Number of observations	References
Skeletal muscle	420 (200–660)	10	27
	36 (0–320)	7	26
	0.12 (0.04–0.19)	2	28
Cardiac muscle	1200 (750–1980)	9	27
	0.27 (0.16–0.38)	2	28
Liver	900	2	29
	710 (360–980)	8	27
	580 (60–1,050)	4	26

Data presented as mean. Numbers in brackets indicate range.

Distribution of Xanthine Dehydrogenase/Oxidase in Skeletal Muscle

The early studies on the localization of xanthine oxidase in human and animal tissues were performed with histochemical techniques and a variety of different distribution patterns were reported [19–21]. In 1981, Jarasch et al. [22] performed the first immunohistochemical examination of xanthine oxidase with the use of polyclonal antibody. These investigators described that xanthine oxidase was located in endothelial cells of microvessels of most tissues, including skeletal muscle, as well as in mammary gland epithelial cells. The localization of the enzyme in endothelial cells of small vessels has also been observed with histochemical techniques [23]. Later immunohistochemical examinations with the use of a monoclonal antibody to xanthine oxidase, also found xanthine oxidase to be present in capillary endothelial cells of skeletal muscle as well as in smooth muscle cells of blood vessels [24]. The two latter studies both reported absence of xanthine oxidase in skeletal muscle cells and in endothelial cells of larger vessels [22, 24]. The presence of the enzyme in capillary endothelial cells of muscle has been confirmed by the demonstration of xanthine oxidase mRNA in this cell type [25].

The activity of xanthine oxidase differs between animal species as well as between tissues and there is also a large discrepancy between reports on the level of xanthine oxidase activities [e.g. 26] (table 1). In general, it appears that the enzyme activity is low in skeletal muscle homogenates, whereas liver holds a relatively high level of activity. It should be pointed out, however, that as the fraction of capillary endothelial cells in muscle homogenate is small, the activity at the actual site of the capillaries is likely to be rather high.

Furthermore, human tissues hold a lower level of activity than for example rat, a difference that should be kept in mind when translating findings from animal studies to the human situation.

Conversion of Xanthine Dehydrogenase to Xanthine Oxidase

In vivo conversion of xanthine dehydrogenase has been demonstrated in a variety of tissues including skeletal muscle, although there is little documentation regarding the mechanisms behind a conversion. McCord [18] and coworkers were originally unable to demonstrate a conversion of xanthine dehydrogenase in rat skeletal muscle subjected to ischaemia, but Lindsay et al. [30] showed that with prolonged ischemia of 5 h, the proportion of xanthine oxidase in canine skeletal muscle increased from 10 to 35%. Similarly, Smith et al. [31] demonstrated that ischaemic rat skeletal muscle had a significantly higher fraction of xanthine oxidase than nonischaemic muscle: 59% versus 30%. Xanthine dehydrogenase has also been shown to be converted to the oxidase form in human skeletal muscle subjected to ischaemia, where conversion to xanthine oxidase occurred when the muscle was kept at room temperature but not when kept at low temperatures [32].

In addition to the proposed possibility of a proteolytic conversion, xanthine dehydrogenase may be converted to its oxidase form via oxidation of critical sulphydryl groups [5]. This could occur via the enzyme sulphydryl oxidase, which is present in tissue such as the liver but which is not thought to be present in skeletal muscle, or in the presence of hydrogen peroxide [33]. The latter mechanism has been shown to occur in perfusion studies, but it is not known whether this occurs in vivo.

A conversion to xanthine oxidase has also been reported to be induced by the presence of immunological mediators. A conversion of xanthine dehydrogenase to its oxidase form has been found in cells and animals subjected to cytokines, such as tumour necrosis factor and the complement C5a [34]. Furthermore, activated neutrophils have been shown to induce the conversion to the oxidase form in endothelial cells in culture [35, 36]. The potential role of xanthine oxidase in inflammation will be discussed in a later section.

We may now raise the question as to whether xanthine dehydrogenase may be converted in the muscle tissue during exercise. A transformation of the enzyme via activated calcium-dependent proteases would require a change in the intracellular calcium homeostasis. Studies on sprinting race horses have shown disturbances of the sarcoplasmic reticulum with consequent abnormal increases in intracellular calcium in the muscle [37]. Highly intensive exercise may also lead to a reduction in adenine nucleotides that possibly could lower the activity of the calcium pumps. However, in order for activated muscle proteases to act on xanthine dehydrogenase localised in the vessel walls, the cell membrane would already have to be disrupted. Alternatively, a conversion to the oxidase form in muscle during exercise could arise via activated proteases within the vascular cells or through other mechanisms, such as oxidation of free sulphydryl groups [5]. The latter mechanism could occur via hydrogen peroxide, but would of course require that this oxygen metabolite was already generated either via xanthine oxidase or via any other source. Finally, with specific exercise conditions, such as following hard eccentric exercise leading to muscle damage, or in a muscle which already suffers from inflammation, conversion of xanthine dehydrogenase to the oxidase form could occur through the presence of immunoparticipating mediators and cells.

Hypoxanthine Formation in Muscle during Exercise

The rate of adenosine 5'-triphosphate (ATP) utilisation during exercise of high intensity can be very rapid and may exceed the rate of ATP regeneration [38, 39]. The concurrent onset of adenosine 5'-diphosphate (ADP) accumulation will lead to increased flux through the adenylate kinase reaction [2 ADP→ ATP + adenosine 5'-monophosphate (AMP)] with the consequence that AMP is formed (fig. 2). AMP does, however, not accumulate in the muscle to a large extent, but is rapidly deaminated to inosine monophosphate (IMP). In contrast to the adenine nucleotides, only a small part of the IMP is further degraded and therefore IMP accumulates in the muscle almost stoichiometrically to the rate of adenine nucleotide degradation [40]. After termination of an intense exercise bout, and possibly also during exercise, IMP is reaminated to AMP in the purine nucleotide cycle whereby the adenine nucleotide pool is restored [e.g. 41, 42] (fig. 2). The alternative fate of IMP is dephosphorylation to inosine via the enzyme purine nucleoside phosphorylase (fig. 2). The flux of IMP through this pathway is rather low in human skeletal muscle, as indicated by a relatively low accumulation of purines in muscle and plasma after intense exercise [43] (fig. 3). The reason for this low rate is probably in part the low activity of purine nucleoside phosphorylase in skeletal muscle homogenates [26]. Nevertheless, some inosine is formed and accumulates in the muscle during exercise. Whereas the cell membrane is more or less impermeable to IMP, inosine can pass through the membrane and enter the blood stream. Inosine can also be further degraded to hypoxanthine, the substrate for xanthine oxidase, which also may pass through the cell membrane. It has been found that hypoxanthine does not accumulate in the muscle during or after intense exercise, despite large increases in muscle IMP [43] (fig. 3), suggesting that hypoxanthine is rapidly released from the muscle after formation. This is supported by findings from studies on purine exchange over intensively excercising muscle where it can be seen that hypoxanthine is released from the muscle (fig. 4). During 90 min of recovery following 45 min of intermittent

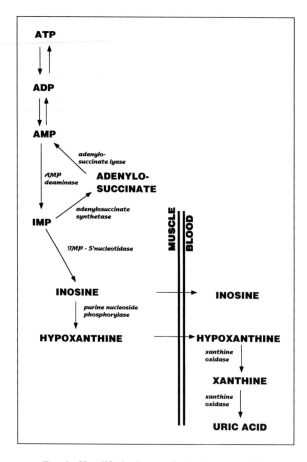

Fig. 2. Simplified scheme of adenine nucleotide metabolism in skeletal muscle.

high-intensity exercise, 150 μmol hypoxanthine has been observed to be released from the exercising leg [Y. Hellsten et al., to be published]. Furthermore, in plasma from subjects that have performed one bout of exhaustive exercise of 2–6 min duration, hypoxanthine is seen to accumulate from about 2 μmol/l in resting value up to 100 μmol/l plasma in some individuals [26].

So what is the fate of hypoxanthine after the release from muscle? As has been discussed, xanthine oxidase appears to be present in the vascular cells of human muscle tissue (table 1) but, despite this fact, it has been observed that the products of hypoxanthine, xanthine and uric acid, are not released from the muscle during and following intensive exercise [44, 45]. Uric acid does nevertheless, accumulate to a large extent in plasma following intense

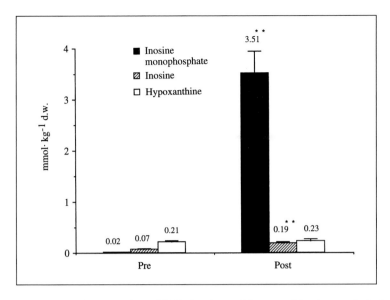

Fig. 3. Concentration of IMP, inosine and hypoxanthine in muscle before and after short-term exhaustive cycling [43].

exercise [46–48], suggesting a main site of uric acid production other than the muscle. The relatively high level of xanthine oxidase activity in the liver would point at this organ as a likely candidate for uric acid formation and in a study where the exchange of purines was measured over the exercising muscle and over the liver, it was found that the liver indeed was releasing uric acid into blood [44]. Hypoxanthine in plasma, originating from the exercised muscle, was extracted and oxidised to uric acid by the liver. Based on estimates from this study, the increase in plasma uric acid after the exercise could almost entirely be attributed to the release from the liver although, as xanthine oxidase has been found present in the capillaries of most tissues [22], it is likely that some of the uric acid in plasma originates from the microvasculature of other organs.

It would appear that as formation of uric acid cannot be detected over the muscle, a significant activity of xanthine oxidase and, thus, the possibility of free radical generation via this enzyme in the muscle would be ruled out. However, firstly, it should be mentioned that the method that has been used for the determination of uric acid release may not be sufficiently sensitive to detect small releases from the muscle. Secondly, uric acid formed in the vascular cells of the muscle may not all be released into the blood. It has been observed that uric acid can be extracted by the exercised muscle, which leaves the

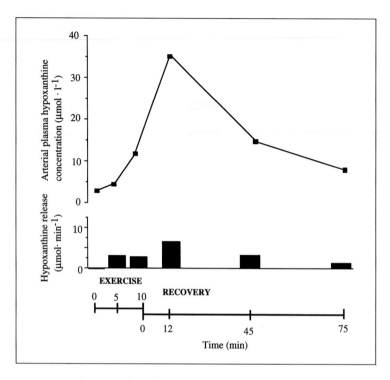

Fig. 4. Concentration of hypoxanthine in plasma (upper panel) and release of hypoxan-thine from muscle (lower panel) during and after 10 min of exhaustive cycling [44].

possibility that uric acid, after being formed in the vascular walls in the muscle, is taken up by the muscle [16, 44] (fig. 5). As will be described later in this chapter, the reason for this uptake may be to scavenge free radicals formed within the muscle.

Is There Evidence for Oxygen-Radical Generation Related to Xanthine Oxidase in Skeletal Muscle?

We will begin with the issue of whether free radicals at all are formed in human muscle during intensive exercise, which would be the most likely type of exercise to metabolically induce free-radical generation via xanthine oxidase. Intermittent sprint training has been found to result in an enhanced activity level of the scavenger enzymes glutathione peroxidase and glutathione reductase in the muscle [26]. As scavenger enzymes act directly or indirectly to remove free radicals, an elevation of these enzymes with training suggests an increased need for free-radical protection. A similar finding was reported by

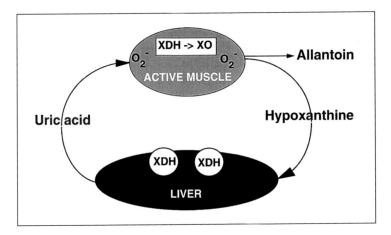

Fig. 5. Schematic representation of the interaction between the exercising muscle and the liver in metabolism of purines. Hypoxanthine formed in the exercising muscle is released into blood. Hypoxanthine is extracted from the blood by the liver which oxidizes the purine to xanthine and uric acid. Uric acid is released from the liver into the blood from where it can be extracted by the exercising muscle for use as a free-radical scavenger.

Oerthenblad et al. [49] where intense jump training was found to lead to a significant increase in the activity of catalase, glutathione peroxidase, gluta-thione reductase and superoxide dismutase in the muscle. In further support of free-radical generation in muscle during intense exercise is the finding that uric acid is non-enzymatically oxidised to allantoin in muscle during short-term exhaustive cycling [16]. This observed oxidation almost certainly occurs due to the presence of free radicals [50, 51], as will be further discussed in the final part of this chapter.

We then arrive at the issue of whether xanthine oxidase may contribute to free-radical generation in skeletal muscle. In the ischaemia/reperfusion model, superoxide radicals are formed when the tissue is again reperfused with oxygen-containing blood, providing xanthine oxidase with the electron acceptor necessary for the oxidation of hypoxanthine formed during the ischaemic phase (fig. 1). By inhibiting xanthine oxidase with specific com-pounds investigators have demonstrated that free-radical generation via xan-thine oxidase is partly responsible for ischaemia/reperfusion-induced muscle damage. Pre-treatment of animals with the xanthine oxidase inhibitors tung-sten or oxypurinol has been found to result in a marked attenuation of the reperfusion-induced increase in vascular permeability in the muscle [52, 53]. Xanthine oxidase has also been found to contribute to lipid peroxidation

[54] and impaired contractile function [55] of rat skeletal muscle subjected to ischaemia/reperfusion. Thus, in this model it appears that xanthine oxidase may play a role in muscle injury.

From the findings described in the first three sections, we may conclude that intensive exercise theoretically provides the requirements for free-radical formation via xanthine oxidase with lowered ATP levels, formation of hypoxanthine and xanthine, and available oxygen, although evidence for the most crucial event, the possible conversion to the oxidase form, is lacking. In theory, a conversion could occur during exercise with high ATP turnover rates, leading to adenine nucleotide degradation, a consequent compromise in the activity of the calcium pumps and an activation of calcium dependent proteases acting on xanthine dehydrogenase. The possibility also exists for a conversion to occur via generation of free radicals, e.g., from the mitochondria, or in the presence of specific immunological substances.

Although the potential may exist, there is only a negligible amount of evidence for xanthine-oxidase-derived free-radical generation in the muscle during exercise. In a study by Duarte et al. [56], xanthine oxidase was reported to be responsible for a decrease in reduced muscle glutathione levels, and morphological changes of exercised muscle in mice [56]. In this study, treatment of the xanthine oxidase inhibitor allopurinol prevented exercise induced mito-chondrial swelling in endothelial cells of muscle. Morphological disturbances of endothelial cells in muscle, which vaguely imply that xanthine oxidase may be involved in damage, have also been observed after long-term endurance exercise [57].

It can be concluded that evidence exists regarding free-radical generation in human skeletal muscle during intensive exercise. However, the indications for xanthine oxidase as a free-radical generator in muscle during exercise are, at this time, hypothetical and more substantial evidence is clearly required to either accept or reject this hypothesis.

Xanthine Oxidase in Inflammation

A physiological explanation for the conversion of xanthine dehydrogenase to its oxidase form with the consequent radical formation has long been sought. Several hypotheses have been put forward where one has been a role of the enzyme in inflammatory processes [10, 58]. This proposition has gained increasing support as an escalating number of studies are demonstrating an interaction between immunological mediators and cells and xanthine oxidase [11, 59–61]. Oxygen metabolites are known to play an important role in biological systems, partly as powerful destructors of microbes but also as mediators

References

1   Chambers DJ, Braimbridge MV, Hearse DJ: Xanthine oxidase as a source of free radical damage in myocardial ischemia. Ann Thorac Surg 1987;44:291–297.
2   Parks DA, Williams TK, Beckman JS: Conversion of xanthine dehydrogenase to oxidase in ischemic rat intestine: A reevaluation. Am J Physiol 1988;254:G768–G774.
3   Lindsay S, Liu T-H, Xu J, Marshall PA, Thompson JK, Parks DA, Freeman BA, Hsu CY, Beckman JS: Role of xanthine dehydrogenase and oxidase in focal cerebral ischemic injury to rat. Am J Physiol 1991;261:H2051–H2057.
4   Della Corte E, Stirpe F: The regulation of rat-liver xanthine oxidase: Activation by proteolytic enzymes. FEBS letters 1968;2:83–84.
5   Della Corte E, Stirpe F: The regulation of xanthine oxidase in rat liver: Modifications of the enzyme activity of rat liver supernatant on storage at –20 °C. Biochem J 1968;108:349–351.
6   Sjödin B, Hellsten-Westing Y, Apple FS: Biochemical mechanisms for oxygen free radical formation during exercise. Sports Med 1991;10:236–254.
7   Smith L: Acute inflammation: The underlying mechanisms in delayed onset muscle soreness. Med Sci Sports Exerc 1991;23:542–551.
8   Diamond JR, Bonventre JV, Karnovsky MJ: A role for oxygen free radicals in aminonucleoside nephrosis. Kidney Int 1986;29:478–485.
9   Linas SL, Whittenburg D, Repine JE: Role of xanthine oxidase in ichemia/reperfusion injury. Am J Physiol 1990;258:F711–F716.
10 Granger DN: Role of xanthine oxidase and granulocytes in ischemia-reperfusion injury. Am J Physiol 1988;255:H1269–H1275.
11 Ghezzi P, Bianchi M, Mantovani A, Spreafico F, Salmona M: Enhanced xanthine oxidase activity in mice treated with interferon and interferon inducers. Biochem Biophys Res Commun 1984;119:144–149.
12 Pfeffer KD, Huecksteadt TP, Hoidal JR: Xanthine dehydrogenase and xanthine oxidase activity and gene expression in renal epithelial cells. J Immunol 1994;153:1789–1797.
13 Becker BF: Towards the physiological function of uric acid. Free Radic Biol Med 1993;14:615–631.
14 Ames BN, Cathcart R, Schwiers E, Hochstein P: Uric acid provides an antioxidant defense in humans against oxidant- and radical-caused aging and cancer: A hypothesis. Proc. Natl Acad Sci USA 1981;78:6858–6862.
15 Smith RC, Lawing L: Antioxidant activity of uric acid and 3-N-ribosyluric acid with unsturated fatty acids and erythrocyte membranes. Arch Biochem Biophys 1983;223:166–172.
16 Tullson P, Bangsbo J, Hellsten Y, Richter EA: Intense, exhaustive exercise in humans decreases muscle uric acid content. Proceedings of the Ninth International Conference on Biochemistry of Exercise, Aberdeen, Scotland, 1994, pp 193.
17 Granger DN, Rutili G, McCord JM: Superoxide radicals in feline intestimal ischaemia. Gastroenterology 1981;81:22–29.
18 McCord JM: Superoxide radical: A likely link between reperfusion injury and inflammation. Adv Free Radic Biol Med 1986;2:325–345.
19 McIndoe WM, Wight PAL, MacKenzie GM: Histochemical demonstration of xanthine dehydrogenase in the tissues of the domestic fowl. Histochem J 1974;6:339–345.
20 Auscher C, Amory N, Pasquier C, Delbarre F: Localization of xanthine oxidase activity in hepatic tissue. A new histochemical method. Int Adv Exp Med Biol 1977;76A:605–609.
21 Sackler ML: Xanthine oxidase from liver and duodenum of the rat. Histochemical localization and electrophoretic heterogeneity. J Histochem Cytochem 1966;14:326–333.
22 Jarasch E-D, Grund C, Bruder G, Heid HW, Keenan TW, Franke WW: Localization of xanthine oxidase in mammary-gland epithelium and capillary endothelium. Cell 1981;25:67–82.
23 Kooij A, Frederiks WM, Gossrau R, Van Noorden CJF: Localization of xanthine oxidoreductase activity using the tissue protectant polyvinyl alcohol and final electron acceptor tetranitro BT. J Histochem Cytochem 1991;39:87–93.
24 Hellsten-Westing Y: Immunohistochemical localization of xanthine oxidase in human cardiac and skeletal muscle. Histochemistry 1993;100:215–222.

25   Räsänen LA, Karvonen U, Pösö AR: Localization of horse mRNA in horse skeletal muscle by in situ hybridization with digoxigenin-labelled probe. Biochem J 1993;292:639–641.
26   Hellsten Y: Xanthine dehydrogenase and purine metabolism in man. With special reference to exercise; thesis, Stockholm, Sweden 1993.
27   Wajner M, RA Harkness: Distribution of xanthine dehydrogenase and oxidase activities in human and rabbit tissues. Biochim Biophys Acta 1989;991:79–84.
28   Watts RWE, Watts JEM, Seegmiller JE: Xanthine oxidase activities in human tissues and its inhibition by allopurinol (4-hydroxypyrazolo [3,4-d]pyrimidine) J Lab Clin Med 1965;66:688–697.
29   Krenitsky TA, Spector T, Hall WW: Xanthine oxidase from human liver: Purification and characterization. Arch Biochem Biophys 1986;247:108–119.
30   Lindsay TF, Liauw S, Romaschin AD, Walker PM: The effect of ischemia/reperfusion on adenine nucleotide metabolism and xanthine oxidase production in skeletal muscle. Vasc Surg 1990;12:8–15.
31   Smith JK, Carden DL, Korthuis RJ: Activated neutrophils increase microvascular permeability in skeletal muscle: Role of xanthine oxidase. J Appl Physiol 1991;70:2003–2009.
32   Wilkins EG, Rees RS, Smith D, Cahmer B, Punch J, Till GO, Smith DJ: Identification of xanthine oxidase activity following reperfusion in human tissue. Ann Plastic Surg 1993;31:60–65.
33   Bindoli A, Cavallini L, Rigobello MP, Coassin M, Di Lisa F: Modification of the xanthine-converting enzyme of perfused rat heart during ischaemia and oxidative stress. Free Radic Biol Chem 1988; 4:163–167.
34   Friedl HP, Till GO, Trentz O, Ward PA: Roles of histamine, complement and xanthine oxidase in thermal injury of skin. Am J Pathol 1989;135:203–217.
35   Phan SH, Gannon DE, Varani J, Ryan US, Ward PA: Xanthine oxidase activity in rat pulmonary artery endothelial cells and its alteration by activated neutrophils. Am J Pathol 1989;134:1201–1211.
36   Wakabayashi Y, Fujita H, Morita I, Kawaguchi H, Murota S: Conversion of xanthine dehydrogenase to xanthine oxidase in bovine carotid artery endothelial cells induced by activated neutrophils: Involvement of adhesion molecules. Biochiem Biophys Acta 1995;1265:103–109.
37   Byrd SK: Alterations in the sarcoplasmic reticulum: A possible link to exercise-induced muscle damage. Med Sci Sports Exerc 1992;24:531–536.
38   Hultman E, Bergström J, McLennan Anderson N: Energy metabolism in single muscle fibres during maximal sprint exercise in man. Scand J Clin Lab Invest 1967;19:56–66.
39   Cheetham ME, Boobis LH, Brooks S, Williams C: Human muscle metabolism during sprint running. J Appl Physiol 1986;61:54–60.
40   Meyer RA, Terjung RL: AMP deamination and IMP reamination in working skeletal muscle. Am J Physiol 1980;239:C32–C38.
41   Löwenstein JM: Ammonia production in muscle and other tissues: The purine nucleotide cycle. Physiol Rev 1972;52:382–414.
42   Tullson PC, Terjung RL: Adenine nucleotide metabolism in contracting skeletal muscle; in Holloszy JO (ed): Exerc Sci Sports Rev. Baltimore Williams & Wilkins, 1991, pp 507–537.
43   Tullson PC, Bangsbo J, Hellsten Y, Richter EA: IMP metabolism in human skeletal muscle after exhaustive exercise. J Appl Physiol: 1995;78:146–152.
44   Hellsten-Westing Y, Ekblom B, Kaijser L, Sjödin B: Exchange of purines in human liver and skeletal muscle with short-term exhaustive exercise. Am J Physiol 1994;266:R81–R86.
45   Sahlin K, Ekberg K, Cizinsky S: Changes in plasma hypoxanthine and free radical markers during exercise in man. Acta Phsiol Scand 1991;142:275–281.
46   Hellsten-Westing Y, Balsom PD, Norman B, Sjödin B, Acta Physiol Scand 1993;149:405–412.
47   Green HJ, Fraser IG: Differential effects of exercise intensity on serum uric acid concentration. Med Sci Sports Exerc 1988;20:55–59.
48   Hellsten-Westing Y, Sollevi A, Sjödin B: Plasma accumulation of hypoxanthine, uric acid and creatine kinase following exhaustive runs of differing duration in man. Eur J Appl Physiol 1991; 62:380–384.
49   Oerthenblad N, Madsen K, Djurhuus S: Muscle and blood antioxidant status and electrolyte homeostasis following supermaximal exercise in trained and untrained humans. Proceedings of the Ninth International Conference on Biochemistry of Exercise, Aberdeen, Scotland, 1994, p 91.
50   Maples KR, Mason RP: Free radical metabolite of uric acid. J Biol Chem 1988;263:1709–1712.

51 Aruoma OI, Halliwell B: Inactivation of a_1-antiproteinase by hydroxyl radicals. The effect of uric acid. FEBS Lett 1989;244:76–80.

52 Sexton WL, Korthuis RJ, Laughlin MH: Microvascular injury after ischemia and reperfusion in skeletal muscle of exercise-trained rats. J Apl Physiol 1990;68:2329–2336.

53 Korthuis RJ, Granger DN, Townsley MI, Taylor AE: The role of oxygen derived free radicals in ischemia induced increases in canine skeletal muscle vascular permeability. Circ Res 1985;57:599–609.

54 Kawasaki S, Sugiyama S, Ishiuro N, Ozawa T, Miura T: Implication of superoxide radicals on ischemia reperfusion induced skeletal muscle injury in rats. Eur Surg Res 1993;25:129–136.

55 McCutchan HJ, Schwappach JR, Enquist EG, Walden DL, Terada LS, Reiss OK, Leff JA, Repine JE: Xanthine oxidase derived H_2O_2 contributes to reperfusion injury of ischaemic skeletal muscle. Am J Physiol 1990;258:H1415–H1419.

56 Duarte JA, Appell H-J, Carvalho F, Bastos ML, Soares JMC: Endothelium derived oxidative stress may contribute to exercise induced muscle damage. Int J Sports Med 1993;8:470–472.

57 Crenshaw AG, Fridén J, Hargens AR, Lang GH, Thornell L-E: Increased technetium uptake is not equivalent to muscle necrosis: Scintigraphic, morphological and intramuscular pressure analyses of sore muscles after exercise. Acta Physiol Scand 1993;148:187–198.

58 McCord JM: Superoxide radical: A likely link between reperfusion injury and inflammation. Adv Free Radic Biol Med 1986;2:325–345.

59 Petrone WF, English DK, Wong K, McCord JM: Free radicals and inflammation: Superoxide dependent chemotactic factor in plasma. Proc Natl Acad Sci USA 1980;77:1159–1163.

60 Diamond JR, Bonventre JV, Karnovsky MJ: A role for oxygen free radicals in aminonucleoside nephrosis. Kidney Int 1986;29:478–485.

61 Adamson GM, Billings RE: The role of xanthine oxidase in oxidative damage caused by cytokines in cultured mouse hepatocytes. Life Sci 1994;55:1701–1709.

62 Terao M, Cazzaniga G, Ghezzi P, Bianchi M, Falciani F, Perani P, Garattini E: Molecular cloning of a cDNA coding for mouse liver xanthine dehydrogenase. Biochem J 1992;283:863–870.

63 Falciani F, Ghezzi P, Terao M, Cazzanigi G, Garattini E: Interferons induce xanthine dehydrogenase gene expression in L929 cells Biochem J 1992;285:1001–1008.

64 Granger DN, Kvietys PR, Perry MA: Leukocyte-endothelial cell adhesion induced by ischemia and reperfusion. Can J Physiol Pharmacol 1993;71:67–75.

65 Grum CM, Gross TJ, Mody CH, Sitrin PG: Expression of xanthine oxidase activity by murine leukocytes. J Lab Clin Med 1990;116:211–218.

66 Hellsten Y, Hansson HA, Johnson L, Sjödin B: Increased presence of xanthine oxidase and insulin like growth factor I (IGF I) in skeletal muscle after a week of strenuous exercise in man. Proceedings of the Ninth International Conference on Biochemistry of Exercise, Aberdeen, Scotland, 1994, p 88.

67 Grum CM, Ragsdale RA, Ketai LH, Simon RH: Plasma xanthine oxidase activity in patients with adult respiratory distress syndrome. J Crit Care 1987;2:22–26.

68 Friedl HP, Smith DJ, Till GO, Thompson PD, Louia DS, Ward PA: Ischemia-reperfusion in humans. Appearance of xanthine oxidase activity. Am J Pathol 1990;136:491–495.

69 Yokoyama Y, Beckman JS, Beckman TK, Wheat JK, Cash TG, Freeman BA, Parks DA: Circulating xanthine oxidase: Potential mediator of ischemic injury. Am J Physiol 1990;258:G564–G570.

70 Adachi T, Fukushima T, Usami Y, Hirano K, Biochem J: Binding of human xanthine oxidase to sulphated glycosaminoglycans on the endothelial cell surface. 1993;289:523–527.

71 Tan S, Yokoyama Y, Dickens E, Cash TG, Freeman BA, Parks DA: Xanthine oxidase activity in the circulation of rats following hemorrhagic shock. Free Radic Biol Med 1993;15:407–414.

72 Cannon JG, Kluger MJ: Endogenous pyrogen activity in human plasma after exercise. Science 1983;220:617–619.

73 Evans WJ, Meredith CN, Cannon JG, Dinarello CA, Frontera WR, Hughes VA, Jones BH, Knuttgen HG: Metabolic changes following eccentric exercise in trained and untrained men. J Appl Physiol 1986;61:1864–1868.

74 Jones DA, Newham DJ, Round JM, Tollfree SEJ: Experimental human muscle damage: Morphological changes in relation to other indices of muscle damage. J Physiol 1986;375:435–448.

75 Round JM, Newham DA, Cambridge G: Cellular infiltrates in human skeletal muscle exercise induced damage as a model for inflammatory muscle disease? J Neurol Sci 1987;82:1–11.

76 Smith LL, McCammon L, Smith S, Chamness M, Israel RG, OBrien KF: White blood cell response to uphill walking and downhill jogging at similar metabolic loads. J Appl Physiol 1989;58:833–837.

77 Hikida RS, Staron RS, Hagerman FC, Sherman WM, Costill DL: Muscle fiber necrosis associated with human marathon runners. J Neurol Sci 1983;59:185–203.

78 Cohen AM, Aberdroth RH, Hochstein P: Inhibition of free radical-induced DNA damage by uric acid. FEBS Lett 1984;174:147–150.

79 Becker BF, Reinholz N, Özçelic T, Leipert B, Gerlach E: Uric acid as a radical scavenger and antioxidant in the heart. Pflügers Arch 1989;415:127–135.

80 Zhong Z, Lemasters JJ, Thurman RG: Role of purines and xanthine oxidase in reperfusion injury in perfused rat liver. J Pharmacol Exp Ther 1989;250:470–475.

81 Wayner DDM, Burton GW, Ingold KU, Barclay LRC, Locke SJ: The relative contributions of vitamin E, urate, ascorbate and proteins to the total peroxyl/radical trapping antioxidant activity of human blood plasma. Biochim Biophys Acta 1987;924:408–419.

82 Maxwell SRJ, Jakeman P, Thomason H, Leguen C, Thorpe GHG: Changes in plasma antioxidant status during eccentric exercise and the effect of vitamin supplementation. Free Radic Res Commun 1993;19:191–202.

Dr. Ylva Hellsten, Copenhagen Muscle Research Centre, August Krogh Institute, Universitetsparken 13, DK–2100 Copenhangen Ø (Denmark)

Marconnet P, Saltin B, Komi P, Poortmans J (eds): Human Muscular Function
during Dynamic Exercise. Med Sport Sci. Basel, Karger, 1996, vol 41, pp 121–133

....

Oxygen Radical Production and Muscle Damage during Running Exercise

Malcolm J. Jackson

Department of Medicine, Muscle Research Centre, University of Liverpool, UK

Introduction

Several studies have indicated the beneficial effects of a moderate amount of exercise on cardiovascular health, but the effects of many years of sustained exercise training and competition on susceptibility to disease in later life or on life span have not been evaluated. Recent data have indicated that an overproduction of oxygen free radicals may be associated with exercise [1, 2] and other workers have proposed that increased free-radical activity may be the cause of ageing [3] and pathogenic for many of the common disorders of old age [4]. Taken together these data may imply that increased free-radical activity during exercise leads to premature ageing and an increased incidence of age-related disorders. It is therefore important to clarify whether free radicals are produced in excess during exercise and to determine the effects and importance of this to the casual and regular athlete.

In recent years, it has also been suggested that the proposed increase in free-radical activity during exercise and the occurrence of muscle damage may be causally related. Muscle pain, together with some loss of force generation, is a common phenomenon following strenuous or unaccustomed exercise in humans [5]. On closer examination these changes may be associated with morphological and ultrastructural disruption of muscle architecture and with the appearance of biochemical markers of muscle damage such as the release of intracellular components (e.g. muscle cytosolic enzymes) into the blood stream.

If it could be demonstrated that this damage is caused by free radicals, this would have major implications for the prevention of muscle damage during training regimens and competitive exercise in athletes and for prevention of exercise-induced muscle pain and damage in sedentary subjects undertaking unaccustomed exercise.

The aim of this review is to critically examine the possible role of oxygen free radicals in muscle damage resulting from different types and duration of running exercise.

Dose Muscle Damage Occur with Running Exercise?

There is little evidence that the more usual forms of running exercise cause substantial muscle damage. Definitive assessment of the extent of muscle damage following athletic events is difficult since this process is most conclusively defined by microscopic examination of muscle. Such investigations require muscle biopsy and, despite the relative lack of trauma involved in modern procedures [6], they have not been frequently undertaken. Most workers have examined the appearance of muscle-specific proteins in the serum or plasma as a less invasive technique for the study of muscle damage in man. These proteins (such as creatine kinase, myoglobin or carbonic anhydrase III) are thought to be released from degrading muscle cells which lose plasma membrane integrity.

Short periods of even very intensive exercise (such as sprinting) do not usually appear to be associated with significant damage to skeletal muscle although some muscle damage is usually reported following long-term exhaustive exercise (such as marathon running). Serum creatine kinase activity appears to peak 24–48 h after these more severe types of prolonged running exercise [7]. More rapid change may occur in other circulating markers of muscle damage such as myoglobin, but overall the data indicate that prolonged endurance exercise can cause a relatively small amount of skeletal muscle damage which is apparent very soon after exercise [8].

A number of studies have now demonstrated that one of the major factors influencing muscle damage following exercise is the predominant manner in which the muscle is used. Muscle may contract in three ways: where the active muscle is allowed to shorten (concentric contractions), remains at fixed length (isometric contractions) or is lengthened (eccentric contractions). Direct comparisons of experimental concentric versus eccentric contractions have demonstrated that repetitive eccentric contractions are much more damaging than concentric contractions [5, 9–12], although the time course of onset of the pain and damage is much slower than seen following excessive concentric contractions. Most standard exercise protocols (e.g. running, cycling etc.) involve a combination of concentric and eccentric contractions with some muscles being used primarily in a concentric and some in an eccentric manner.

Occasional forms of exercise, such as predominantly down hill running, involve extensive use of a number of muscles in an eccentric manner and, are therefore very damaging to muscle tissue.

It is therefore clear that running can cause damage to skeletal muscle although it is necessary for the event to be either of a prolonged nature or for the predominant muscular activity to involve lengthening contractions for substantial muscle damage to occur.

Free Radicals in Muscle

A free radical can be defined as a species capable of independent existence that contains one or more unpaired electrons. The unpaired electron confers charge on the particle and because the electron is dynamic, the species exhibits a magnetic charge – and is termed paramagnetic. The unpaired electron is depicted conventionally as a dot, e.g. the hydroxyl radical is $OH^{\bullet}$. Usually, O_2 undergoes 6-electron reduction with the generation of H_2O. However, 1-electron reduction of O_2 (that is receipt of one electron) produces superoxide $(O_2^{\bullet-})$. If 2-electron reduction occurs and 2 hydrogen atoms are donated H_2O_2 (hydrogen peroxide) is formed. Iron and copper demonstrate variable valency, in that they readily fluctuate between valency states by donating/receiving electrons (e.g. Fe^{2+} (ferrous) which has two electrons less than ground state and Fe^{3+} (ferric) which has three less).

This ability to receive and donate electrons makes possible the catalysis of a number of reactions as in the presence of hydrogen peroxide (the Fenton reaction):

$$Fe^{2+} + H_2O_2 \rightarrow Fe^{3+} + OH^{\bullet} + OH^-$$

$$Fe^{3+} + H_2O_2 \rightarrow Fe^{2+} + O_2^{\bullet-} + H^+$$

Iron is also capable of catalysing the production of hydroxyl radicals from the peroxide radical:

$$Fe^{3+} + O_2^{\bullet-} \rightarrow Fe^{2+} + O_2$$

$$Fe^{2+} + H_2O_2 \rightarrow Fe^{3+} + OH^{\bullet} + OH^-$$

the net result is:

$$O_2^- + H_2O \rightarrow O_2 + OH^{\bullet} + OH^-$$

(the iron-catalysed Haber-Weiss reaction) [13].

This is postulated to be an extremely important mechanism in biology – since the superoxide radical is relatively unreactive, but its production in enzymic reactions could lead to production of $OH^{\bullet}+OH^-$ which may damage important molecules in the cell. In the aqueous-phase superoxide mainly acts as a reducing agent and produces hydrogen peroxide. However, as has been seen, in the presence of a catalyst such as iron the much more reactive hydroxyl radical could be formed.

Due to their reactive nature free radicals are capable of damaging a number of biological substances:

(a) Membrane lipids: Oxygen-derived radicals have been shown to be capable of damaging membrane-bound cholesterol [14] and fatty acids by the process of lipid peroxidation. This was first appreciated following the absorption of air by walnut oil in the last century by de Saussure, and its subsequent rancidification. The abstraction of a hydrogen atom from a polyunsaturated fatty acid produces the fatty acid radical. This arrangement is unstable and following molecular rearrangement during which there is a change in the steric configuration from the *cis* to the *trans,* the more stable conjugated diene is formed, which now has double bonds separated by a single carbon. This has characteristic UV absorption properties which make it useful as a marker of free-radical activity. Following the uptake of oxygen and the formation of the peroxy radical the reaction may proceed as a autolytic chain reaction, producing the lipid hydroperoxide or the lipoperoxide free radical. Fragmentation of the molecule may then occur to produce aldehydes, such as malonaldehyde (a marker of free-radical activity) which may further react with amino groups from adjacent proteins to produce fluorescent lipid peroxidation products which are also readily measurable [15].

(b) Protein oxidation: Denaturation of proteins by cross-linkage and fragmentation may be induced by hydrogen peroxide, implicating hydroxyl radicals [16] and effects on immunoglobulin by free radicals have also been observed [17]. Collagen and hyaluronic acid damage can be caused by superoxide and it has been suggested that this may play a major role in the pathogenesis of certain inflammatory disorders [15, 18].

(c) DNA: Strand breakage has been observed following exposure of DNA to superoxide [19, 20] and free radicals have been implicated as having a role in the DNA-damaging effects of certain drugs [21].

Sources of free radicals in muscle: Free radicals are recognised to be formed as a by-product of normal metabolism and it has been suggested that the increased oxygen consumption by exercising muscle tissue must lead to increased oxygen-radical production by mitochondria [22]. However, a comparison of the damage which occurs during eccentric compared with concentric activity of muscle and the relative changes in oxygen consumption in these

Table 1. Possible sites for oxygen radical production in muscle during exercise

---

Primary sources
1   Mitochondrial electron transport chain
2   Xanthine oxidase activity
3   Prostanoid metabolism
4   Membrane-bound oxidase activity,
       e.g. NAD(P)H oxidase

Secondary sources
5   Phagocytic white cells
6   Secondary to muscle calcium accumulation
7   Secondary to disruption of iron-containing proteins

Xanthine oxidase may not be found within skeletal muscle tissue, but is found in the vascular endothelium closely associated with muscle tissue. Data from Sjodin et al. [22], Bendich [24] and Jackson [23].

---

situations [23] illustrates that such an increase cannot be the only explanation for exercise-induced muscle damage. A number of other potential intracellular and extracellular sites for oxygen-radical production during exercise have been suggested [22–24], but their importance is unclear. Potential sites of oxygen-radical production during exercise are presented in table 1, these are divided into sites which may produce oxygen radicals as primary initiators of the degeneration of biomolecules and sites where radicals may be produced secondary to degeneration. A major problem in the assessment of the role of free radicals in any situation is whether they are a primary or secondary to the initial damaging process [25].

Evidence for Increased Production of Free Radicals during Exercise

The unequivocal demonstration of increased free radical activity in complex biological tissues is difficult and is usually only accepted if a variety of indicators provide supportive evidence. This can be in the form of measurements of indirect indicators of free radical activity (products of lipid peroxidation, DNA oxidation, protein oxidation), direct detection of free radicals (electron spin resonance techniques) or prevention of the putative free-radical-mediated effect by supplementation with relatively specific anti-oxidants.

Initial suggestions that free-radical processes, such as lipid peroxidation, were elevated during exercise came from studies of whole-body exercise in man [2] and rats [26, 27]. These were rapidly followed by studies of the products of free-radical reactions within the tissues of exercising animals [1]. These data indicated that exercise to exhaustion in rats resulted in decreased mitochondrial respiratory control, loss of sarcoplasmic reticulum integrity, increased lipid peroxidation and increased free-radical generation as shown by electron spin resonance studies. This is the most widely quoted data paper supporting a role for free-radical species in exercise-induced damage to skeletal muscle (and other tissues). It is notable that the exercise regimen used was an endurance protocol in which the muscles were primarily contracting in a concentric manner.

Various indicators of free-radical-mediated lipid peroxidation appear to be elevated in muscle from exercising animals [1, 26, 27] and man [2]. Contractile activity of skeletal muscle is associated with an increase in an electron spin resonance signal derived from free-radical species in muscle [1, 28], and with a loss of glutathione from the tissue [29, 30]. Gohil et al. [29] have suggested that glutathione is oxidised in muscle and rapidly transported from muscle to blood for reduction at non-muscle sites, thus providing a shuttle of reduced glutathione for the exercising muscle. Data from exercising humans are in general agreement with his proposal [31, 32] (fig. 1). In studies of the heart, Ferrari et al. [33, 34] and Curello et al. [35] have demonstrated that there is an oxidation of intracellular glutathione during ischaemia and concluded that the extent of this oxidation is an important determinant of the vulnerability of the heart to damage during reperfusion. Our studies in skeletal muscle do not support such a crucial role for glutathione in contraction-induced damage [30].

Repeated periods of exercise reduce the likelihood of damage to skeletal muscle during subsequent bouts of the same form of exercise and this appears to be associated with an increase in the activity of muscle superoxide dismutase [36], a reduced level of lipid peroxidation products during exercise in trained rats [37], and a modification of the concentration of antioxidants and activity of antioxidant enzymes in trained humans [38]. Quintanilha and Packer [39] and Packer [40] have also examined the exercise endurance of animals of modified antioxidant capacity and found that vitamin-E-deficient rats have a reduced endurance capacity, while Amelink [41] has reported that vitamin-E-deficient rats have an increased amount of injury following treadmill exercise.

The concept has therefore arisen that, during high-intensity oxidative exercise, the increased formation of oxidising free radicals (probably of mitochondrial origin) can damage muscle tissue, and that training regimens or antioxidant supplementation may reduce this by elevating muscle antioxidant capacity.

Table 2. Changes in contractile properties of triceps surae after 60 min box stepping

	Placebo	Vitamin C-treated	Vitamin E-treated
MVC (N)			
Rest	1,118 (82)	1,223 (76)	1,201 (93)
After exercise	855 (67)	987 (66)	882 (41)
20/50 Hz			
Rest	0.73 (0.01)	0.78 (0.02)	0.75 (0.03)
After exercise	0.41 (0.04)	0.59 (0.05)*	0.47 (0.04)

*Significantly increased compared with placebo-treated subjects. Data from Jakeman and Maxwell [63].

There is also some support for the concept that free radicals play a role in post-exercise fatigue of muscle. Initial studies reported that 'spin-trapping' agents and vitamin E prolonged the exercise endurance of swimming mice [42], although these authors did not attempt to differentiate whether their results were due to an effect on muscle damage or fatigue. Careful studies of the diaphragm have now been undertaken to look for evidence of free-radical involvement in fatigue of this muscle. Shindoh et al. [43] demonstrated a protective effect of N-acetylcysteine against diaphragm fatigue in rabbits in vivo when fatigue was induced by repetitive electrical stimulation of strips of the diaphragm in situ. N-acetylcysteine was reported to reduce the onset of both low- and high-frequency fatigue, but did not improve the rate of recovery from either. These results are somewhat surprising in that previous data have indicated that different mechanisms underlie low- and high-frequency fatigue. Following cessation of contractile activity, most studies have indicated that high-frequency fatigue reverses rapidly, whereas the force deficit apparent at low frequencies persists for considerably longer [44]. Some data indicate that high-frequency fatigue is likely to be due to changes in intracellular and extracellular ion concentrations, while low-frequency fatigue is secondary to an abnormality in excitation-contraction coupling [43]. The protective effects of N-acetylcysteine against the onset of both forms of fatigue are therefore difficult to explain. It is possible that a common free-radical-mediated mechanism mediates both types of fatigue and that this is inhibited by N-acetylcysteine, or that oxidation of protein sulphydryls is common to both processes and inhibited by N-acetylcysteine. However, it is also entirely possible that N-acetylcysteine acted indirectly by improving the delivery of substrates (such as oxygen or glucose) to the exercising muscle.

More direct support for a role of free-radical species in the mechanisms underlying diaphragm fatigue was provided by Reid et al. [45, 46]. They studied fibre bundles from rat diaphragm in vitro and demonstrated an apparent increase in intracellular [45] and extracellular [46] oxidant formation during contractile activity. Various antioxidant substances (catalase, SOD and di-methyl sulphoxide) were also found to inhibit the onset of low-frequency fatigue, although no effects on high-frequency fatigue were observed.

These data are therefore in general support of the hypothesis that free-radical species contribute to the genesis of muscle fatigue. The interpretation of these latter data is however, complicated by the use of isolated bundles of fibres from the diaphragm as a model system. Such preparations are inherently unstable and lack longer-term viability because of the trauma to muscle fibres occurring during dissection of the strips or bundles of fibres. Effects of antioxidants might therefore reflect improved preservation of tissue viability rather than effects on the fatigue process. In an attempt to clarify this position, we have studied the effect of antioxidants of fatigue in an isolated rodent skeletal muscle system [47], but have been unable to confirm the reported effects of antioxidants.

Eccentric exercise has been infrequently studied from the point of view of free-radical processes, but where damage to skeletal muscle specifically induced by eccentric contractions has been studied, conflicting data have been reported [48]. Saxon et al. [49] studied the effects of either repetitive lengthening or shortening contractions of the knee extensors in man and found that lengthening contractions damaged muscle, but neither protocol influenced significantly indirect markers of free-radical activity. In contrast, others have reported that exercise which primarily involves lengthening contractions is associated with increases in indirect measures of free radical activity [50].

Do Free Radicals Mediate the Muscle Damage Caused by Excessive Running Exercise?

Whether free radicals cause muscle damage following various types of running exercise can only be firmly ascertained by intervention studies. Vitamin E appears to be the antioxidant which has received most attention in terms of potential use to reduce exercise-induced oxidative stress. Early workers in this field examined the effect of vitamin E depletion on the amount of lipid peroxidation [26] and the free-radical signal visible by electron spin resonance

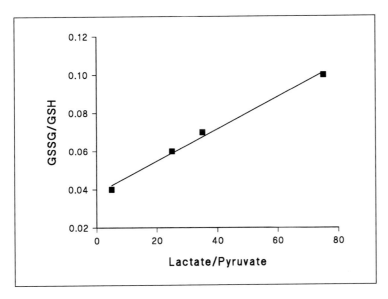

Fig. 1. Relationship between whole blood oxidised/reduced glutathione and lactate/pyruvate ratio following exercise. Data from Sastre et al. [32].

[1] in exercising muscle, and found that vitamin-E-depleted animals had evidence of increased free-radical activity associated with a reduction in exercise endurance. These effects of antioxidant depletion on exercise endurance were confirmed by further studies from the same group [40] and exacerbatory effects of vitamin E deficiency on other models of exercise-induced muscle damage were reported by Jackson et al. [51] and Amelink [41].

Our group has specifically examined the effects of vitamin E on damage processes in isolated skeletal muscle. These studies have demonstrated that vitamin E has protective effects against contractile activity-induced [51, 52] and calcium-ionophore-induced [53–55] damage to skeletal muscle in vitro, but the mechanisms by which this protective effect occurs do not appear to be as clear-cut as some workers have proposed. Although the protective effects are apparent in animals fed diets rich in polyunsaturated fatty acids, but not in animals fed a diet rich in saturated fatty acids [56], data which are in general agreement with the concept that the excess vitamin E is preventing free-radical-mediated peroxidation of membrane polyunsaturated fatty acids, the protective effects also appear to be mimicked by phytol, osophytol and a number of other lipophilic, non-antioxidant substances having long hydrocarbon side chains [53, 55]. It is therefore clear that further work is required in this area to clarify the nature of the protection offered by vitamin E.

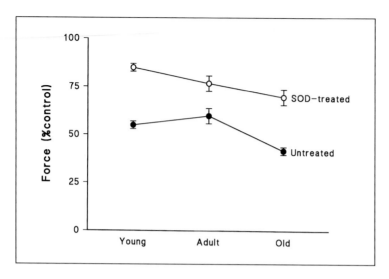

Fig. 2. Effect of SOD treatment on the force deficit in mice of different ages at 3 days following a protocol of lengthening contractions. Redrawn from Zerba et al. [58].

All of these preceding studies were undertaken in exercise models where the predominant form of muscle activity was not specified or where it was entirely isometric. Eccentric exercise has been infrequently studied from the point of view of free radical processes, but where damage to skeletal muscle specifically induced by eccentric contractions has been studied, conflicting data have been reported. In a detailed study of damage to mouse extensor digitorum longus muscle induced by eccentric contractions, Zerba et al. [58] found that treatment of animals with polyethylene glycol superoxide dismutase significantly reduced the amount of injury which was present 3 days after exercise in mice of various ages (fig. 2). However, in a study of animals undertaking lengthening contractions during downhill walking, Warren et al. [57] could show no protective effect of vitamin E supplementation. Cannon et al. [59] have also examined subjects undertaking downhill running. They found no protective effects of vitamin E supplementation against muscle damage although the supplements did appear to reduce oxidative stress [60] and these authors suggest that their data support a role for oxidants in delayed-onset muscle damage.

Other antioxidants have only been infrequently studied as potential inhibitors of the deleterious effects of exercise, but those data which have been presented are inconclusive concerning possible protective effects of these substances [24, 32, 61]. However, in a recent study, Jakeman and Maxwell

[62] studied the effects of vitamin C on eccentric exercise in man and reported a reduced low-frequency fatigue after exercise in the treated subjects (table 2).

Conclusion

It is clear that there is now substantial evidence in support of an increased production of free-radical species during running exercise, but the evidence that these species are responsible for any skeletal muscle damage which occurs as a result of the exercise is much less conclusive. It is also clear that training enhances the antioxidant capacity of muscle, but whether antioxidant nutrient supplements are beneficial to subjects undertaking excessive or unaccustomed exercise is still not clearly established.

References

1   Davies KJA, Quintanilha AT, Brooks GA, Packer L: Free radicals and tissue damage produced by exercise. Biochem Biophys Res, Commun 1982;107:1198–1205.
2   Dillard CJ, Litov RE, Savin WM, Tappel AL: Effects of exercise, vitamin E and ozone on pulmonary function and lipid peroxidation. J Appl Physiol 1978;45:927–932.
3   Harman D: A theory of ageing based on free radicals and radiation chemistry. J Gerontol 1956; 11:298–3-5.
4   Halliwell B, Gutteridge JMC: Free Radicals in Biology and Medicine, ed. 2. Oxford, Clarendon Press, 1989.
5   Newham DJ, Mills KR, Quigley BM, Edwards RHT: Pain and fatigue after concentric and eccentric muscle contractions. Clin Sci 1983;64:55–62.
6   Dietrichson P, Coakley J, Smith PEM, Griffiths RD, Helliwell TR, Edwards RHT: Conchotome and needle percutaneous biopsy of skeletal muscle. J Neurol Neurosurg Psychiatry 1987;50:1461–1467.
7   Noakes TD: Effects of exercise on serum enzyme activities in humans. Sports Med 1987;4:245–267.
8   Roxin LE, Hedin G, Venge P: Muscle cell leakage of myoglobin after long-term exercise and relation to the individual performances. Int J Sports Med 1980;7:259–263.
9   Newham DJ, Jones DA, Edwards RHT: Plasma creatine kinase changes after eccentric and concentric contractions. Muscle Nerve 1986;9:59–63.
10 Newham DJ, Jones DA, Tolfree SEJ, Edwards RHT: Skeletal muscle damage: A study of isotope uptake, enzyme efflux and pain after stepping. Eur J Appl Physiol 1986;55:106–112.
11 Armstrong RB: Muscle damage and endurance events. Sports Med 1986;3:370–381.
12 Armstrong RB: Initial events in exercise-induced muscular injury. Med Sci Sports Exerc 1990;22: 429–435.
13 Cotton A, Wilkinson A: Advanced Inorganic Chemistry. New York, Wiley, 1987.
14 Smith I: Cholesterol Autoxidation. New York, Plenum Press, 1981.
15 Halliwell B, Gutteridge JMC: Free Radicals in Biology and Medicine, Oxford, Clarendon Press, 1985.
16 Wolff S, Garner A, Dean R: Protein denaturation by hydrogen peroxide. Trends Biol Sci 1986;11: 27–31.
17 Hewitt S, Lunec J, Morris C, Blake D: Effect of free radical altered IgG on allergic inflammation. Ann Rheum Dis 1987;46:866–874.

18 Greenwald R, Moy W, Lazarus D: Degradation of cartilage proteoglycans and collagen by superoxide radical. Arthritis Rheum 1976;19:799.

19 Brawn K, Fridovitch I: DNA strand scission by enzymically generated oxygen radicals. Arch Biochem Biophys 1981;206:414–419.

20 Ward J, Burton G, Ingold K: Radiation and hydrogen peroxide-induced free radical damage to DNA. Br J Cancer 1986;55:105–112.

21 Quinlan G, Gutteridge J: Oxygen radical damage to DNA by rifamycin 5V and copper ions. Biochem Pharmacol 1987;36:3629–3633.

22 Sjodin B, Westing YM, Apple FS: Biochemical mechanisms for oxygen free radical formation during exercise. Sports Med 1990;10:236–254.

23 Jackson MJ: Exercise and oxygen radical production by muscle; in Sen CK, Packer L, Hanninan O (eds): Exercise and Oxygen Toxicity. Amsterdam, Elsevier, 1994, pp 49–57.

24 Bendich A: Exercise and free radicals: Effects of antioxidant vitamins. Med Sports Sci 1991;32: 59–78.

25 McArdle A, Jackson MJ: Intracellular mechanisms involved in damage to skeletal muscle. Basic Appl. Myology 1994;4:43–50.

26 Brady PS, Brady LJ, Ulrey DE: Selenium, vitamin E and the response to swimming stress in the rat. J Nutr 1979;109:1103–1109.

27 Gee DL, Tappel AL: The effect of exhaustive exercise on expired pentane as a measure of in vivo lipid peroxidation in the rat. Life Sci 1981;28:2425–2429.

28 Jackson MJ, Edwards RHT, Symons MRC: Electron spin resonance studies of intact mammalian skeletal muscle. Biophys Acta 1985;847:185–190.

29 Gohil K, Viguie CA, Stanley WC, Packer L, Brooks GA: Blood glutathione oxidation during human exercise. J Appl Physiol 1988;64:115–119.

30 Jackson MJ, Kaiser K, Brooke MH, Edwards RHT: Glutathione depletion during experimental damage to rat skeletal muscle and its relevance to Duchenne muscular dystrophy. Clin Sci 1991; 80:559–564.

31 Duthie GG, Robertson JD, Maughan RJ, Morrice PC: Blood antioxidant status and erythrocyte lipid peroxidation following distance running. Arch Biochem Biophys 1990;282:73–83.

32 Sastre J, Asensi M, Gasco E, Pallardo FV, Ferrero JA, Furakawa T, Vina J: Exhaustive physical exercise causes oxidation of glutathione status in blood: Prevention by antioxidant administration. Am J Physiol 1992;263:R992–R995.

33 Ferrari R, Ceconi C, Curello S: Oxygen-mediated myocardial damage during ischaemia and reperfusion: Role of the cellular defences against oxygen toxicity. J Molec Cell Cardiol 1985;17:937–945.

34 Ferrari R, Curello S, Ceconi C, Cargoni A, Condorelli E, Albertini A: Intracellular effects of myocardial ischaemia and reperfusion: Role of calcium and oxygen, Eur Heart J 1986;7(suppl A): 3–12.

35 Curello S, Ceconi C, Cargnoni A, Connacchian A, Ferrari R, Albertini A: Improved procedure for determining glutathione in plasma as an index of myocardial oxidative stress. Clin Chem 1987;33: 1448–1449.

36 Higuchi M, Cartier LJ, Chen M, Holloszy JO: Superoxide dismutase and catalase in skeletal muscle: Adaptive response to exercise. J Gerontol 1985;40:281–286.

37 Alessio HM, Goldfarb AH: Lipid peroxidation and scavenger enzymes during exercise: Adaptive response to training. J Appl Physiol 1988;64:1333–1336.

38 Robertson JD, Maughan RJ, Duthie GG, Morrice PC: Increased blood antioxidant systems of runners in response to training load. Clin Sci 1991;80:611–618.

39 Quintanilha AT, Packer L: Vitamin E, physical exercise and tissue oxidative damage; in Porter R, Whelan J (eds): Biology of Vitamin E. Ciba Foundation Symposia Series No 101. London, Pitman, 1983, pp 56–69.

40 Packer L: Vitamin E, physical exercise and tissue damage in animals. Med Biol 1984;62:105–109.

41 Amelink GJ: Exercise induced muscle damage, PhD thesis, Utrecht, 1990.

42 Novelli GP, Bracciotti G, Falsini S: Spin trappers and vitamin E prolong endurance to muscle fatigue in mice. Free Radic Biol Med 1990;8:9–13.

43 Shindoh C, Dioharco A, Thomas A, Manubray P, Supinski G: Effect of N-acetylcysteine on diaphragm fatigue. J Appl Physiol 1990;68:2107–2113.
44 Gibson H, Edwards RHT: Muscle exercise and fatigue. Sports Med 1985;2:120–132.
45 Reid MB, Haack KE, Franchek KM, Valberg PA, Kobzik L, West MS: Reactive oxygen in skeletal muscle. I. Intracellular oxidant kinetics and fatigue in vitro. J Appl Physiol 1992;73:1797–1804.
46 Reid MB, Shoji T, Moody M, Entman ML: Reactive oxygen in skeletal muscle. II. Extracellular release of free radicals. J Appl Physiol 1992;73:1805–1809.
47 Jackson MJ, McArdle A, O'Farrell S: Free radicals, muscle fatigue and muscle damage; in Blake DR, Winyard PC (eds): Immunopharmacology of Free Radical Species. New York, Academic Press, 1995, pp 175–182.
48 Jackson MJ, O'Farrell S: Free radicals and muscle damage. Br Med Bull 1993;49:630–641.
49 Saxon JM, Donnelly AE, Roper HP: Indices of free radical-mediated damage following maximum voluntary eccentric and concentric muscular work. Eur J Appl Physiol 1994;68:189–193.
50 Packer L, Viguie C: Human exercise: Oxidative stress and antioxidant therapy; in Benzi G (ed): Advances in Biochemistry. 2. Libbey Eurotext, London, 1989, pp 1–17.
51 Jackson MJ, Jones DA, Edwards RHT: Vitamin E and skeletal muscle; in Porter R, Whelan J (eds): Biology of Vitamin E. Ciba Foundation Symposia Series No. 101. London, Pitman, pp 224–239.
52 McArdle A, Edwards RHT, Jackson MJ: Calcium homeostasis during contractile activity of vitamin E-deficient skeletal muscle. Proc Nutr Soc 1993;52:83A.
53 Phoenix J, Edwards RHT, Jackson MJ: Inhibition of calcium-induced cytosolic enzyme efflux from skeletal muscle by vitamin E and related compounds. Biochem J 1989;257:207–213.
54 Phoenix J, Edwards RHT, Jackson MJ: Effects of calcium ionophore on vitamin E deficient rat muscle. Br J Nutr 1990;64:245–256.
55 Phoenix J, Edwards RHT, Jackson MJ: The effect of vitamin E analogues and long hydrocarbon chain compounds on calcium-induced muscle damage. A novel role for α-tocopherol. Biochim Biophys Acta 1991;1097:212–218.
56 O'Farrell S, Jackson MJ: Unpublished observations.
57 Warren JA, Jenkins RR, Packer L, Witt EH, Armstrong PB: Elevated muscle vitamin E does not attenuate eccentric exercise-induced muscle injury. J Appl Physiol 1992;72:2168–2175.
58 Zerba E, Komorowski TE, Faulkner JA: Free radical injury to skeletal muscles of young, adult and old mice. Am J Physiol 1990;258:C429–C435.
59 Cannon JG, Orencole SF, Fielding RA, Meydani M, Meydani SN, Fiatrone MA, Blumberg JB, Evans WJ: Acute phase response in exercise: Interaction of age and vitamin E on neutrophils and muscle enzyme release. Am J Physiol 1990;259:R1214–R1219.
60 Meydani M, Evans WJ, Handelman G, Biddle L, Fielding RA, Meydani SN, Burrill J, Fiatrone MA, Blumberg JB, Cannon JG: Protective effect of vitamin E on exercise-induced oxidative damage in young and older adults. Am J Physiol 1994;264:R992–R998.
61 Gerster H: The role of vitamin C in athletic performance. J Am Coll Nutr 1989;8:636–643.
62 Jakeman P, Maxwell S: Effect of antioxidant vitamin supplementaation on muscle function after eccentric exercise. Eur J Appl Physiol 1993;67:426–430.

Prof. Malcolm J. Jackson, Muscle Research Centre, Department of Medicine,
University of Liverpool, PO Box 147, Liverpool L69 3BX (UK)

Marconnet P, Saltin B, Komi P, Poortmans J (eds): Human Muscular Function during Dynamic Exercise. Med Sport Sci. Basel, Karger, 1996, vol 41, pp 134–147

....

Neuromuscular Fatigue in Stretch-Shortening Cycle Exercises

Caroline Nicol [a], *Paavo V. Komi* [b]

[a] Movement and Perception, Faculty of Sport Sciences, University of the Mediterranean, Marseille, France
[b] Department of Biology of Physical Activity, University of Jyväskylä, Finland

Natural forms of over-ground locomotion make use of active repetitive stretch-shortening cycles (SSC) of lower-limb extensor muscles [1]. SSC muscle actions are characterized by a powerful final shortening action that is known to rely partly on the recoil of elastic energy and on the assistance of stretch reflexes. However, exhaustive SSC exercises may lead to ultrastructural muscle damage, which is usually associated with gradually developing muscle soreness and inflammation [2] and a long-lasting decline in maximal isometric force [3]. Reductions in the efficacy of the SSC muscle action have also been reported at the end of short-lasting [4] as well as long-lasting [5] exhaustive SSC exercises. In these studies, the parallel analysis of the vertical ground reaction forces indicated reduced tolerance to impact. This may be expected to result from the induced contractile failure as well as from a lesser intervention of the stretch reflexes to stiffness regulation.

The present report will focus on the underlying mechanisms that could contribute to the functional defects and delayed recovery usually observed after SSC-type exercise. After a brief review of the characteristics of this type of fatigue, the question of the neuromuscular changes and/or adaptations to fatigue will be discussed quite extensively with greater emphasis on the reflex modifications in case of SSC fatigue.

Characteristics of Stretch-Shortening Cycle Fatigue

Many exercises, especially unaccustomed strenuous activities, can result in muscle damage and functional defects. SSC-type exercises combine eccentric and concentric muscle actions and the induced fatigue corresponds clearly to that reported after the eccentric ones. During the last 20 years, there has been increasing interest in how eccentric muscle actions lead to delayed-onset muscle soreness (DOMS) and/or tissue damage [for reviews, see ref. 6, 7].

Description of the Muscle Damage

Delayed, but reversible, ultrastructural muscle damage is a good indicator of injury resulting from exercises involving eccentric muscle action. Following long-lasting runs, histological examinations have revealed muscle fibre necrosis and breakdown associated with accumulations of mitochondria, erythrocytes, leucocytes and phagocytes within the muscle fibres [2]. Shorter but more intensive exercise consisting of downstairs running was found to induce marked broadening, streaming and even total disruptions of the myofibrillar Z-band [8]. In some reports, however, little or no damage has been observed in the biopsy samples. This was the case, for instance, after a 100-km running competition [9]. Referring to some animal studies, this could result partly from the fact that the muscle lesions could be localized within specific muscles and not homogeneously distributed throughout the muscle fibres [10]. In addition, Fridén et al. [11] recently revealed the presence of subtle intracellular changes of eccentrically exercised muscles, that would not be generally detected by routine histological stainings. However, it seems logical that the skeletal muscle can adapt to repeated eccentric exercise, but this adaptation process with concomitant disappearance of soreness may last up to 2 weeks [12].

Serum Enzyme Levels as Indicator of Muscle Fibre Damage

The presence of enzymes in the blood that are normally localized in muscle fibres is considered as an indicator of increased permeability or disruption of the muscle cell membranes [for reviews, see ref. 7, 13]. As creatine kinase (CK) is found almost exclusively in muscle tissue, serum or plasma CK is the most commonly used marker of muscle damage. It should be noted, however, that due to the considerable variability of the magnitude of the response of serum enzymes [14] the measured CK peak level does not reflect the amount of muscle damage.

Potential Causes and Mechanisms of Morphological Damage

It has been demonstrated that muscle injury, as indicated by increased levels of muscle-specific enzymes in the blood, increases with the intensity and duration of the exercise [15], and lasts for several days. Armstrong [16] differentiates four stages in the progressive process. The 'initial stage' (I) includes the events that trigger the whole process. The 'autogenetic stage' (II) corresponds to the first 3–4 h after-injury and marks the beginning of the degrading process of the membrane structures. The 'phagocytic stage' (III) is characterized by a typical inflammatory response in the tissue which may last for 2–4 days or more. The 'regenerative stage' (IV) begins on days 4–6 and reflects the regeneration of muscle fibres. By days 10–14, the injured muscle appears usually normal. The present focus will be on potential mechanisms that may underlie the first 3 stages.

In pure eccentric work, much evidence exists that the initial local damage results from mechanical strain rather than from metabolic mechanisms [17]. The metabolic hypothesis, which refers to 'metabolic overload' and electrolyte accumulation, is refuted by the fact that eccentric muscle actions require less energy and less EMG activity [18] than concentric muscle actions. This of course, applies for comparable force levels, but in case of maximum contraction the activation levels are the same in eccentric and concentric actions [19]. Thus evidence is available that a given tension can be generated across a reduced number of recruited fibres under eccentric conditions [17]. This tension may thus be considered as great enough to lead to the reported subcellular mechanical damage. In prolonged SSC exercises, this possibility is strengthened by the considerable number of ground impacts and eccentric muscle actions encountered. In a recent study, Lieber and Fridén [20] suggested, however, that it is not high force per se that causes damage, but the magnitude of the active strain.

The 'autogenetic stage' of the next 3–4 h could rely more on metabolic changes such as increase of free O_2 radical production and lipid peroxidation [21]. In addition, intracellular accumulation of Ca^{2+} is likely to occur during intensive exercise and to cause potential lesions to the sarcolemma [22]. Such metabolic mechanisms are not, however, specific to either eccentric- or SSC-type exercises.

The characteristic inflammation of the subsequent 'phagocytic stage' has been extensively studied, but the underlying mechanisms are not yet clearly understood. Referring to Fantone [23] and Evans and Cannon [7], it appears that the inflammatory response begins with changes in the vascular wall structure, leading to alterations of the structure and function of the basement membrane and leakage of plasma components to the extravascular tissue. This plasma extravasation produces the clinical sign of oedema and provides a fresh supply of mediators which could partly explain the prolonged duration of the inflammation.

Delayed-Onset Muscle Soreness

DOMS is the sensation of pain and discomfort that increases in intensity in the first 2 days after the exercise, remaining symptomatic for 1 or 2 more days, and disappearing usually 5–7 days after the exercise [see review in ref. 24]. Sore muscles are often stiff or tender, and their ability to produce force is reduced for several days or weeks [3, 25]. At first, discomfort is mostly present in the distal and lateral regions of the exercised muscles, but later it appears to progress to other compartments [26].

Although the delayed onset of stiffness parallels the onset of delayed muscle swelling, the degree of ultrastructural damage does not correlate well with the DOMS intensity [25]. Soreness is not either constant all the time, being mostly felt when the exercised limbs are extended or fully flexed or when the muscles are palpated deeply [25].

Soreness Perception

When peripheral tissues are damaged, the sensation of pain in response to a given stimulus is enhanced. This phenomenon, termed 'hyperalgesia', may involve a lowering of threshold of nociceptors by the presence of locally released chemicals [6]. Hyperalgesia can occur both at the site of tissue damage and in the surrounding undamaged areas [for a review, see ref. 28]. The sensation of pain in the skeletal muscles is transmitted by nociceptors that belong to two different groups of small-diameter group III and IV muscle afferents [29, 30]. They are particularly dense in the regions of connective tissues, but also between intra- and extrafusal muscle fibres as well as near blood vessels, in the Golgi tendon organs and at the myotendinous junction. More specifically, group III carries sharp, localized pain, whereas group IV carries dull and diffuse pain. Group IV fibres have been suggested by Armstrong [31] to be primarily responsible for the sensation of DOMS.

In addition to peripheral pathways, exercise-induced soreness appears to be modulated at the spinal level by the reticular activating system or by the sensory cortex [32]. Variation in receptor types and the ability to modulate pain at multiple levels in the nervous system could partly explain the intersubject variability in soreness perception. In addition, evidence exists of descending influences on the transmission of the sensory afferent information via the spinocervical tract [33, 34]. These observations raise the question of potential interactions between muscle damage, muscle activation and stretch-reflex regulation.

Training Effects on Muscle Damage and Delayed-Onset Muscle Soreness

A beneficial effect of either eccentric [35] or SSC [36, 37] training has been suggested from the measurement of a diminished circulating CK activity after subsequent repetitions of the same exercise. A single bout of intensive eccentric exercise [38] has been shown to attenuate also the DOMS felt during the subsequent bouts of exercise performed within the next 6 weeks.

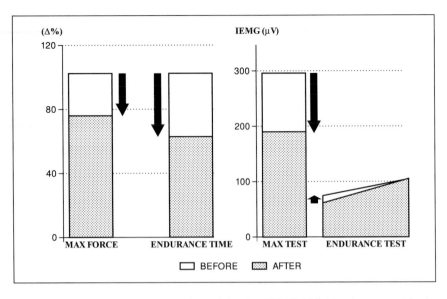

Fig. 1. Relative performance (left) and absolute IEMG (right) levels measured in the maximal and endurance isometric tests performed before and after the marathon run. Modified from Nicol et al. [40].

Combined Effects of Stretch-Shortening Cycle Exercises on Neuromuscular Function

In the following references are made to some of our studies on the SSC-induced fatigue effects on the contractile force and the α-motoneuron pool activation as well as on the SSC muscle action. The reports are in logical consequence for our earlier publications on the topic [4, 39]. Special emphasis will be put on the adaptations of the reflex loops to the induced contractile failure.

Influence on Neural Activation and Force Production

The isometric strength tests can be used reliably to investigate the effects of SSC exercise on the neuromuscular function. Dramatic declines in maximal isometric force have been demonstrated after both long-lasting and short but intensive periods of SSC exercises. In a recent marathon [40], the induced $26 \pm 14\%$ loss in maximal force of the quadriceps muscle group was accompanied by a clear decline ($39 \pm 9\%$) in the capacity to maintain a 60% submaximal isometric level of force (fig. 1 left). The parallel analysis of the electromyographic activity revealed a large decrease in maximal activity ($p < 0.05$), but also the need for an initial increase of the neural activation at

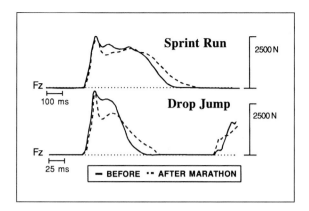

Fig. 2. Group-averaged vertical (Fz) ground reaction force-time curves of two successive sprint contacts and two DJs recorded before and after marathon. Modified from Nicol et al. [5].

submaximal force level, which is likely to indicate a deterioration of the muscle function (fig. 1 right). These observations support the assumption of a contractile failure, and suggest modifications of the neural activation to compensate for it. The isometric tests indicate a facilitation at submaximal force level and an inhibition in maximal force condition.

Influence on Stretch-Shortening Cycle Type Performances

In the same marathon study, contractile failure and changes in the neural activation were detected also in the SSC-type performances [41]. In addition to a 16% decline in either sprint run or drop jump (DJ) tests, the before-after marathon comparison of the ground reaction force-time curves revealed a clear drop in the vertical force after the impact peak with a concomitant increase of the contact time (fig. 2). These observations are well in agreement with the GRF changes reported after a shorter but more intensive SSC exercise [4]. The kinematic behavior of the lower extremity in the pre- and post-marathon treadmill runs indicated similar trends and thus reflect an attempt of the nervous system to compensate for reduced elastic recoil by increased work during the push-off phase. The observed loss of tolerance to impact raises the problem of the effect of fatigue on the stretch-reflex contribution to the reflex regulation.

Influence on the Refex Sensitivity

In order to examine further the effects of SSC exercise on stretch-reflex sensitivity, two studies were performed, in which a stretch reflex test of the shank muscles was performed in a more controlled situation of passive stretches.

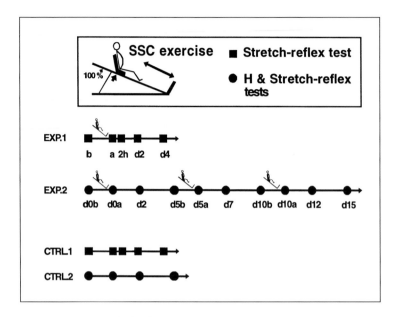

Fig. 3. Chronological representation of the testing protocols performed by the experimental (EXP) and control (CTRL) sessions during the two fatigue experiments. (b = before the sledge exercise; a = after the sledge exercise; 2h = 2 h later; d0–15 = 0–15 days later).

In both studies, fatigue was induced on a sledge apparatus by performing as many rebounds as possible to a given rising height (70% of the maximum). On the average, exhaustion was reached after 100–400 repetitions, i.e. after 2–5 min of intensive work. As shown in figure 3, the potential influence of fatigue on reflex sensitivity was investigated in the first study [42] immediately before and after the sledge exercise, as well as 2 and 4 or 5 days later. In the second experiment [43], the whole protocol was repeated successively 3 times, on days 0, 5 and 10. Each experiment included a control session, in which the subjects performed only the reflex tests. In both experiments, the stretch-reflex test of the shank muscles was performed in a sitting position with the knee stabilized at 120° (fig. 4). A powerful engine was used to induce stretches of the shank muscles at either 70 or $115° \cdot s^{-1}$. This test included a randomized series of 20 mechanical stimuli per velocity. Reflex latency and peak-to-peak amplitude were measured for each recorded reflex and then averaged per velocity. In the second experiment, the reflex tests included both stretch- and H-reflex measurements of the soleus muscle (16 stimuli, 25% maximal M-wave). In this case, the pedal was fixed so that the ankle angle was kept at 90°. Blood concentration of lactate and serum creatine kinase activity were

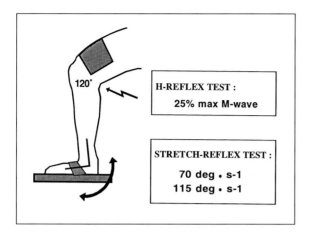

Fig. 4. Schematic representation of the stretch and H-reflex tests used in the various fatigue experiments.

measured at various moments along the protocol. Two maximal drop jumps were also performed after each reflex test.

The analysis of the sledge exercise indicated a significant 5–7% increase ($p < 0.05$) of the contact time towards the time of exhaustion. The EMG analysis revealed a significant $44 \pm 31\%$ reduction ($p < 0.05$) of the lateral gastrocnemius (LG) preactivation. Time to exhaustion did not differ significantly between the 3 tests on the sledge on the second experiment. The before-after fatigue comparison of the stretch-reflexes (fig. 5) revealed an immediate decrease of the peak-to-peak reflex amplitude in both experiments. This was accompanied in the second experiment by a significant reduction ($p < 0.05$) of the H-reflex over M-wave ratio. On the other hand, no significant changes were found in either reflex latency (39 ± 2 ms) or duration. The subsequent analysis of the follow-up period revealed similar trends in both experiments with a significantly delayed recovery of the peak-to-peak stretch reflex amplitude after the sledge exercise. As shown in figure 6, the repetition of the sledge exercise on days 5 and 10 further delayed the reflex recovery. In the case of the H-reflex, the stimulus was not mechanical and did thus not rely on muscle spindle sensitivity. The respective changes of the H- and stretch-reflex amplitudes were positively related on the 5th day after exercise ($r = 0.91$ at $70° \cdot s^{-1}$ and $r = 0.90$ at $115° \cdot s^{-1}$, $p < 0.05$). In the first experiment, the decrease in amplitude was accompanied on day 2 by an absence of 20% of the LG responses at the slowest stretching velocity.

From the metabolic analysis, similar mean peak lactate values (11–15 $mmol \cdot l^{-1}$) were found after the 3 sledge exercises. The serum level of CK

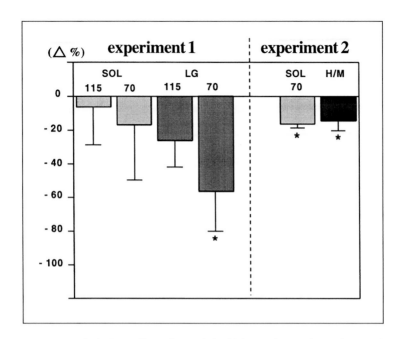

Fig. 5. Left: Immediate effects of the SSC exercise on the peak-to-peak stretch-reflex amplitude of the soleus (SOL) and lateral gastrocnemius (LG) in response to two different stretching velocities (115 and 70 ∘ s^{-1}). Right: Respective effects on the H reflex over M-wave ratio of the SOL muscle. The relative group average values ($\pm$SD) are expressed in percentage change of the initial results. *p < 0.05 signifies comparisons between the experimental and control groups.

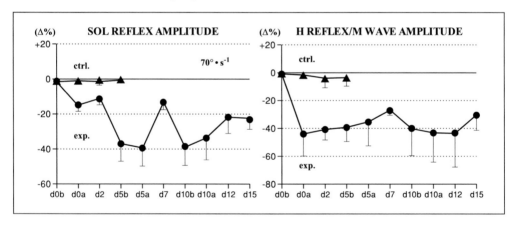

Fig. 6. Relative group-averaged changes ($\pm$SD) of the soleus peak-to-peak stretch-reflex amplitude at 70 ∘ s^{-1} (left) and H reflex over M-wave ratio (right) induced by three successive exhaustive sledge exercises (performed on d0, d5 and d10). Modified from Nicol et al. [43].

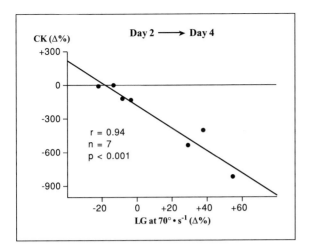

Fig. 7. Relationships between the individual changes measured between the 2nd and the 4th day after exercise in the relative values of serum CK activity and mean LG reflex amplitude in the series of stretches at $70 \circ s^{-1}$.

presented the characteristic pattern observed after repeated eccentric muscle actions, with an essentially individual, but clearly delayed peak of accumulation, which occurred in each experiment on day 2. It should be noted that only part of the subjects returned to their initial CK level on days 4 or 5. The perceived soreness developed usually as soon as 2 h after the exercise and lasted until day 4 in most of the subjects. Furthermore, in the first experiment, the increase in CK activity between the 2nd hour and the 2nd day after exercise was negatively related to the respective changes in DJ height ($p < 0.001$), so that large increases in the relative CK activity were associated with a further decrease in DJ performance. The subsequent decrease in the relative CK activity between days 2 and 4 was significantly related ($p < 0.05$) to the recovery of the relative peak-to-peak reflex amplitude of the LG (fig. 7).

The present results indicate an immediate reduction and delayed recovery of the reflex loop sensitivity after exhaustive SSC exercise. This contrasts with the increased reflex sensitivity reported by another SSC fatigue study [44]. Referring to the study of Gollhofer et al. [39], it is suggested that the contradictory results of these studies could be attributed to the possibility that the neuromuscular system may adapt differently depending on the fatigue level and requested task. The complexity of the reflex changes with fatigue is also illustrated by the studies of Duchateau and Hainaut [45], in which fatigue induced by electrostimulation resulted in a reduction in H-reflex amplitude, whereas the long-latency reflex amplitude was clearly increased. Regarding the present reduction, it may be expected to result from two major and not mutually exclusive processes: (1) a reduction of the excitatory input (disfacilitation) from the muscle spindles [46] and (2) an increased inhibition originating from the sensitization of small-diameter muscle afferents [47]. Regarding the first hypothesis, it has been observed in mammalian muscle that the spindle activity can be reduced and even suppressed at low intracellular pH [48]. Although supported by the present peak lactate values, this possibility is attenuated by the parallel decrease of the H- over M-ratio; a reflex loop which does not involve the muscle spindle. According to Mense and Meyer [49], a reduced sensitivity of muscle spindle to stretch could also result from some of the chemical agents that are directly released from the damaged muscles.

The hypothesis of a reflex inhibition of the input through the sensitization of small-diameter muscle afferents has been suggested by various studies, in which fatigue was induced either by isometric work [50, 51] or by electrostimulation [52, 47]. Group III [3] and group IV [29] nerve endings have been demonstrated to be sensitive to intracellular increases in potassium, phosphate or lactate as well as to low pH, which are known to accompany sustained intensive exercises. Kniffki et al. [29] suggested that the changes induced by normal muscular exercise may not constitute effective stimuli. In case of muscle damage, however, biochemical substances such as bradykinin are released, which enhance the activity of some nociceptors [52]. On the perceptual side there is a prolongation of the pain sensation long after the termination of the stimulus. In this line, most of the present subjects reported long-lasting sensations of muscle pain and discomfort after the sledge exercise. It is therefore suggested that the sensitization of small muscle afferents to both chemical and mechanical processes related to muscle damage could partly explain the delayed recovery of the stretch- and H-reflex sensitivites. This hypothesis is reinforced by the significant relationship that was found in the first experiment between the recovery of the serum CK activity and reflex sensitivity (fig. 7). This inhibition could partly also explain the loss of 20% of the stretch-reflex response at the slowest stretching velocity. Referring to the significant correlation between the increase in serum CK activity and the decline in DJ during the first 2 days, it is suggested that a potential decrease of the stretch reflex sensitivity could have affected the muscle stiffness and, consequently, SSC function.

In conclusion, these findings support the hypothesis that intensive SSC exercise may lead to immediate decrease and delayed recovery of the stretch-reflex sensitivity, which could explain partly the parallel decline in SSC performance. It is suggested that this delayed recovery could result mostly from the indirect influence of muscle damage, via the development of inflammation and muscle soreness, on the sensitization of small diameter afferents.

Subject Index

Mechanical power output
  aging effects 17–19
  growth effects 17
  maximum power in humans
    contributions from muscle fiber types
      11, 12
    mechanical efficiency and shortening
      velocity 12, 14
    oxygen consumption relationship 14
    sustaining power output 12, 14, 15
    voluntary measurement 10, 11
  measurement with isokinetic cycle
    ergometer 10, 21
  velocity of shortening relationship 3, 5–8
Metabolic energy consumption,
  measurement 57, 58
Metabolism, repeated high-energy exercise
  effects 21, 22
Muscle
  damage from running 122, 123, 128–131
  fiber composition
    adaptation in man 86, 88–91
    determination 90
    endurance versus power athletes 88
  force-velocity relationship 82, 83
  plasticity
    acute 15, 17
    chronic 15
  stretch-shortening cycle, see
    Stretch-shortening cycle
  velocity of shortening
    ATP concentration effects in anaerobic
      conditions 1
    effects on efficiency in aerobic conditions
      3, 5–8
    evolutionary considerations 8
    maximum in humans 11, 12, 14
    measurement in dog gastrocnemius 2
    mechanical power output relationship
      3, 5–8
    myosin isoforms 84
    oxygen consumption relationship 3–8
    rate and efficiency of contraction 1, 2
    switching in animal models 85, 86
Myosin
  isoforms
    disuse effects 91, 92
    shortening velocity 84
    training effects 88–91

  types 83, 84
  structure 82

Oxygen consumption
  measuring 49, 50
  metabolic energy consumption calculation
    57
  power output relationship 14
  repeated intense exercise 27–29
  running economy, see Running velocity
    of shortening relationship 3–8

Power output, see Mechanical power output

Reactive oxygen species
  aging role 121
  antioxidant defense systems 96–99, 104
  biological damage 95, 96, 121–123
  Fenton reaction 123
  Haber-Weiss reaction 123
  muscle fatigue role 127, 128
  production in exercise 95, 100, 103, 104,
    121, 125–128
  sources in muscle 124, 125
Running
  economy variation in individuals 33, 58
  energy cost of running
    body size relationship 35–37
    calculation 33, 57, 58
    effect on athletic performance 40
    energy production relationship 62–64
    experimental measurement 34, 35,
      60–68
    sex influence 38–40
    sprinting 35
    training effects 37, 38, 41
  mechanical efficiency
    kinematic arm method 61–64
    measurement 60, 61
    spring mass model 65–68
    stretch-shortening cycle 54, 59, 60
  mechanical work paradox 59, 60
  muscle damage mechanisms 122, 123
  treadmill design for force measurements
    66, 67

Shortening velocity, see Muscle
Stretch-shortening cycle
  defined 44

fatigue
  creatine kinase as marker 135, 141, 143, 144
  delayed-onset muscle soreness 136, 137
  effects
    force production 138, 139
    neural activation 138, 139
    performance 139
    reflex sensitivity 139–141, 143, 144
  induction 140
  mechanisms 136
  muscle damage 134, 135
  soreness perception 137
  stages 135, 136
force-length curves 46
force-velocity curves 46, 47
measurement 45, 46
mechanical efficiency
  measuring 47–50, 52–54
  running 54, 59, 60
  stretching velocity relationship 50
  training effects 50
Superoxide dismutase
  effects of exercise 126
  muscle damage prevention 130
Surface electrical stimulation
  commercial instrumentation 72
  rehabilitation therapy 71
  research applications 71, 72
  training application
    amplitude of stimulation 74
    discomfort minimization 79
    endurance training 76, 78
    mechanism of benefits 78
    muscle growth 77
    outcome 76–78
    power athletes 76–78
    pulse duration 72, 73, 76
  voluntary effort comparison
    fiber activation 74, 75
    force development 75, 76
    motor units recruitment 73, 74

Training
  effects
    antioxidant defense systems 97–99
    delayed-onset muscle soreness 137
    energy cost of running 37, 38, 41
    muscle fiber type adaptation 88–91
    stretch-shortening cycle 50
  surface electrical stimulation
    amplitude of stimulation 74
    discomfort minimization 79
    endurance training 76, 78
    mechanism of benefits 78
    muscle growth 77
    outcome 76–78
    power athletes 76–78
    pulse duration 72, 73, 76
Treadmill
  design for force measurements 66, 67
  evaluation of energy cost of running 34, 35

Uric acid
  free radical scavenging 104, 114–116
  production in exercise 108–110

Vitamin C
  effect of training 99
  effect on muscle fatigue 131
Vitamin E
  effect of training 99
  effect on endurance 126, 127
  muscle damage prevention 128–130
  supplementation 100

Xanthine oxidase
  conversion from xanthine dehydrogenase 106, 107, 112, 113, 116
  distribution in skeletal muscle 105, 106, 116
  exercise enhancement 113, 114
  forms 102
  free radical generation 103, 104, 110–112
  inhibitors 111
  reactions catalyzed 102, 103
  role
    inflammation 112–114, 116
    muscle injury 111, 112